D1592900

Dear Doctor: It's About SEX...

Dear Doctor:
It's About
SEX...

Dr. Lawrence E. Lamb

Walker and Company
New York

First published in the United States of America in 1973
by the Walker Publishing Company, Inc.

Published simultaneously in Canada by Fitzhenry &
Whiteside, Limited, Toronto.

ISBN: 0-8027-0397-6

Library of Congress Catalog Card Number: 72-83117

Printed in the United States of America

Contents

I	Sex Is, Always Was, and Ever Shall Be	1
II	Doing What Comes Naturally	13
III	Special Problems of Women	45
IV	Birth Control and Abortions	66
V	Sterility	101
VI	Masturbation	117
VII	Homosexuality, Male and Female	134
VIII	Impotence and Related Problems	152
IX	Female Sexual Dysfunction	173
X	Male Anatomy Problems	191
XI	Breasts	205
XII	Menopause—Male and Female	224
XIII	Female Surgery	242
XIV	The Prostate Gland	257
XV	Sex in Later Years	272
XVI	Discharge and Hygiene	287
XVII	Venereal Disease	293
XVIII	A Question of Clothing	314
XIX	Miscellaneous Sex Questions	327

Acknowledgment

JUST TWENTY-FIVE YEARS AGO it would not have been possible to write this book. As Alfred Kinsey discovered when students asked questions about sex there were very few objective answers. Without the information that has since been gathered, many of the people's problems presented in this book would have had to be approached using concepts dating back to the birth of Christ. Kinsey correctly observed that our society operated "under a system of sex law which is basically the Talmudic Code of the seventh century B.C." The early pioneers in sexual research have made my job of dealing with the many questions about sex from readers of my syndicated medical column possible and I have depended heavily upon their important contributions in preparing these answers.

One of the first modern pioneers in these areas from the United States was Dr. Robert L. Dickinson. His work was especially important in relation to sexual anatomy and the physiology of the female reproductive system. The reader of this book will see a number of quotes taken from his studies.

Dickinson's early work was followed by the monumental works of Dr. Alfred Kinsey and his collaborators. In more recent times Dr. William Masters and Virginia Johnson have added much needed objective information on what actually happens during sexual activity and on important problems in sexual dysfunction. I am indebted to their valuable work for information which has helped to answer many of my readers' questions.

Then I have relied upon the standard medical references and texts of physiology, psychiatry, urology, obstetrics, and gynecology. The recent monthly publication of *Medical Aspects of Human Sexuality* for physicians and other scientists has been an invaluable source of information, including interesting historical items that shed much light on the history of sexual behavior.

These various sources of information have made it possible for me to deal with people's sexual problems in the same objective manner I would with a patient's problems with any other organ system such as the heart and circulation. The doctor's goal is to help people with their problems, not to pass moral judgments, and it matters little whether the patient's discomfort is the result of mental anguish or physical pain. It requires an objective approach as free as possible from personal prejudices or moral hangups—in short, the scientific way. It is necessary to deal with problems on the basis of facts, not on what one imagines is morally right or wrong. The data from research over the past twenty-five years have done much to make this possible.

I would also like to express my appreciation to Robert Metz, president and editor of Newspaper Enterprise Association for his encouragement to answer my column readers' many letters on these subjects in book form. The Newspaper Enterprise Association's medical column made it possible for me to collect a library of people's problems which I used to prepare this book.

L.E.L., M.D.

Texas, 1973

I

Sex Is, Always Was, and Ever Shall Be

"UNFORTUNATELY IN THE YELLOW PAGES of the telephone book the answer can't be found. At least I have not discovered it. Where do you go to discuss problems in sex? Yes, this common day word has got the best of me."

This was the beginning of one of the thousands of letters I have received about sex. Since I began writing a daily medical column read by several million people in all walks of life, I have come face to face with the real problems people have with one of the most important aspects of their lives—sex. But since in reality we are not face to face, people feel less constraint and tell me their hopes, fears, and deepest secrets. I am the faceless friend to whom they can write without the embarrassment of personal contact. Many a letter writer states frankly that he would be embarrassed to discuss his problem with his doctor and is writing to me for help out of sheer desperation. What follows is the written "cry for help" that reveals what really concerns the individual. He bares his anguish on a piece of paper and more often than not signs it.

The letters are far more eloquent than simple statistics on sexual problems, such as the frequency of impotence or the problems of frigidity. They record the stories of real people and their most intimate lives. the theoretical problems of marriage manuals fall away to be replaced by the reality of life told as it really is. And frequently the secret so carefully

1

protected is the same one that another reader is also worrying about.

We are doing better. The idea that sex is a secret is gradually disappearing in our society. The tremendous mass of individuals seeking fundamental information on sex as it applies to the essential aspects of their daily living is a healthy sign.

Changes in attitude toward sexuality have made sex information available in many ways. Despite my reader's remarks, in some areas you can obtain sex information via the telephone. In New York City there is a Community Sex Information and Education Service, telephone number 212-867-9044. This service tries to answer the questions that people have about sex. Their line is usually busy.

Despite the evidence of improved knowledge and understanding, there are areas in which we have lost ground rather than progressed. To illustrate, venereal disease has had a resurgence in the United States and in much of the world to levels unequaled since World War II. In the United States gonorrhea is the second most common contagious disease, exceeded only by the common cold. Syphilis is on the rise. Despite the advances that have been achieved in medicine and the fact that venereal disease for a time had nearly disappeared, it is now a major problem of our society, affecting all age groups and social strata. Many authorities feel that the sharp rise in venereal disease is a direct outgrowth of two P's—the pill and permissiveness.

A second evidence of lack of progress is the sharp rise in the number of unwed mothers. The tragedy of the young teen-age girl, pregnant and without a mate, is a grim picture. There are many, less obvious, aspects of understanding our sexual life that have shown very little progress. Masters and Johnson (Dr. William H. Masters and Virginia E. Johnson, authors of *Human Sexual Response and Human Sexual Inadequacy*) believe that over half of all American marriages suffer from some form of sexual dysfunction. Many of these dysfunctions are never acknowledged or identified, and thus are not corrected. People are reluctant to tell their problems

2

even to their doctor. A vehicle for truly ascertaining the nature of sexual activity and the problems that can surround it is difficult to find within our society.

Not all forms of sexual activity are simply reflex actions. Much about sex has to be learned. With the change in our society it has become increasingly important for people to learn about sex. Not so long ago a major portion of the population of the United States lived on farms or in small towns within farming communities. This direct contact with nature provided children an immediate example of the nature of sex.

Despite the popular phrase, people learned about sex from animals other than the "birds and the bees." This indeed is fortunate since the anatomy and behavior of birds is quite a bit different from mammals, and the sexual history of the bees is enough to deter any male. (The drone, or male bee, who engages in sexual activity has one glorious fling: he flies off with his queen to the sky and expires after his sexual escapade.) A large portion of our younger people today do not have the opportunity to see a calf born or to see the normal events of the sexual cycle within the setting of nature. Thus one of the best teaching examples possible to educate younger people about natural sex has been lost to most.

In sex, as with other things, our value judgments are often restricted to our own narrow sphere of experience. Thus it is within Judeo-Christian societies that a sexual code for behavior, or morality, has been developed that is unique specifically to those societies. It is hard for us to realize that these sets of values may have little meaning to individuals reared in other cultural backgrounds. Moral judgments in our society may not be applicable to another society. To assume that we are right and all other societies are wrong in all aspects is an inflexible attitude, to say the least.

The sexual behavior in a given society is dictated by the moral code, taboos, and sometimes myths of that society. Ofttimes it may have little or nothing to do with the natural sexual instincts and behavior of the individual. In short, people are conditioned to certain sexual attitudes. These are

3

sometimes in conflict with our fundamental human drives.

The code or values of society can indeed affect the sexual behavior of people. There is no better example of this than the history of sex in England and the United States. The Victorian age assumed sex was to be enjoyed by the male, and submitted to by the female. In that age a British doctor, William Acton, spread his gospel that women had no sexual desire and to state otherwise was "a vile aspersion." In the United States the Surgeon General of the Army, William Hammond, stated flatly that "decent" women did not experience pleasure in bed.

Some of these ideas no doubt had their origin in the concept that sex was bestial or dirty. Part of this concept may well be tied to the obvious fact that the sexual organs are anatomically related to the elimination of excrement. Many societies have believed that excrement included evil spirits and that the process of elimination cleansed the body of poison and evil. Regardless of its origins, the dictum that women were sexless resulted in many women being just that —sexless. They would rather be ladies and conform to the image society held for ladies than to enjoy their normal physical responses. Fortunately, women have largely been liberated from the illusions of the Victorian age. Nevertheless this example in history points up the enormous influence that a society's attitude can have upon the form of sexual behavior of the individual.

Even a casual perusal of the history of man and his behavior within different cultural settings demonstrates that people are capable of almost any form of sexual activity. By our standards there are many extremes in sexual behavior in other cultures. In the Waghi Valley of New Guinea the natives live in an Eden-like setting, literally a paradise filled with well-ordered gardens. But in these primitive people an enormous hostility exists between men and women. The boys are taken from their mothers when they are seven years of age to live with their fathers. Their genitals are scarified at puberty, supposedly to rid them of their mother's blood. The concept of male superiority is carried to the point that the

4

man pierces his mate's thigh with an arrow preceding his one-night visit.

However, the male is not always the dominant partner. The hostility of women toward men is exemplified by the Amazons of Greek mythology. The likelihood that Amazon tribes existed gained strength recently with the observations of a probable Amazon civilization within the rain forests of Brazil. Jesco Von Puttkamer, a German ethnologist, found evidence, including drawings in secret caves, that gives credence to the existence of an Amazon society. Among the evidence was a copulation rock where it is presumed that the Amazon warriors took their male prisoners for fornication. It has been hypothesized that one basin which was found was used for the sacrifice of any male babies.

It is not necessary to return to Greek mythology or antiquity to find examples of sexual behavior that are at variance with what is at least acknowledged within our society. For example, both men and women confined to a prison environment frequently engage in homosexual activity. Evidence indicates the isolation of one of the sexes commonly results in this form of sexual expression.

Two extremes of sexual behavior within different cultures are exemplified by the lives of Nero and Gandhi. Nero exemplified the undisciplined personality who gave his passions full reign, undeterred by social restraint. He progressed from a youth undistinguished by his sexual exploits to a man who engaged in almost every conceivable form of sexual excess. He seduced married women, free-born boys, and finally raped the Vestal Virgin Rubria. It is said that after he rode in curtained vehicles with his mother, he stepped forth with his clothes in disarray, having just engaged in incest. Finally he had the young boy Sporus castrated in an effort to turn him into a girl, then married him in a ceremony attended by all his court with his castrate attired in a bridal veil.

Gandhi, on the other hand, followed the Hindu idea that manly vigor, health, and longevity were dependent upon sexual continence. To this end he renounced his wife and lived a life of celibacy. The Hindus believe that semen is necessary

5

for the vitality of the mind and body. Gandhi was the epitome of sexual self-discipline. However he did find solace in being held by naked women. When associates reproved him for this act he explained that to be rocked by a naked woman and remain unaroused was a test of his will.

In the Judeo-Christian society the thought of sex between the young and old is unacceptable. Yet in other cultures the young boys are introduced to the mysteries of sex by the older women, while the young girls are introduced to sexual activity by the older men. Thus the older generation accepts the responsibility of passing on their knowledge and experience in one of life's most vital areas to the next generation, just as they do other aspects of living.

There are an infinite variety of different practices within different cultures related to sexual activity. In preparation for the wedding night the pubic hair may be removed from the prospective bride by the other women of the wedding party. Still another tribal custom is the amputation of the vulva of the female, presumably with the intention of decreasing her "unclean sexual desire." The men do not necessarily escape either. One tribal custom includes the slitting of the urethra from the tip to the base of the penis. It is not too surprising that many young men approaching the manhood ritual run away from their tribe rather than face this initiation ceremony. The concept of marriage differs greatly within different cultures. In some societies a wife exists solely for the purposes of providing legal heirs, while sexual pleasure is found elsewhere; in others a man might have several wives or even a harem; and the Eskimos have a tradition of offering one's wife to an honored guest, a practice totally unacceptable in much of the Judeo-Christian civilization.

Prostitution is regarded differently from society to society with some cultures honoring it, others, such as the United States, considering it a disgrace. Yet the sale of sex in one form or another has been part of man's experience for centuries. A philosophical point can be made for the observation that the woman who sells herself in marriage for economic gain and social standing is engaging in nothing more

6

nor less than socially acceptable prostitution. Prostitution still flourishes in its strictest definition, and if the simple definition of sex for sale in or out of marriage is applied, it is an almost universal daily experience.

One way of learning what people can and will do is to look at the laws and taboos that are set up to regulate a society. Laws are set up to prohibit acts which people are apt to perform. Thus there are laws against stealing because people do steal. One can gain an idea of the range of human activity that people are capable of by looking at the ancient book of commandments by Moses Maimonides, a famous Jewish scholar of the twelfth century. His writings also shed light on the basis of many of the concepts of morality which have been handed down in the Judeo-Christian society. Among the list of negative commandments it is forbidden:

To have intercourse with one's mother
To have intercourse with one's father's wife
To have intercourse with one's sister
To have intercourse with the daughter of one's father's wife if she be his sister
To have intercourse with one's son's daughter
To have intercourse with one's daughter's daughter
To have intercourse with one's daughter
To have intercourse with a woman and her daughter
To have intercourse with a woman and her son's daughter
To have intercourse with a woman and her daughter's daughter
To have intercourse with one's father's sister
To have intercourse with one's mother's sister
To have intercourse with the wife of one's father's brother
To have intercourse with one's son's wife
To have intercourse with a brother's wife
To have intercourse with a sister of his wife during the latter's lifetime
To have intercourse with a menstruating woman
To have intercourse with another man's wife
For men to lie with beasts
For women to lie with beasts

For a man to lie carnally with a male
For a man to lie carnally with his father
For a man to lie carnally with his father's brother
To be intimate with a kinswoman
To have intercourse without marriage

Efforts toward helping people better understand themselves and sex have resulted in sex education in schools. This is met with responses ranging from enthusiastic acceptance to outright rejection and hostility by parents. Even Sunday school has become a setting for sex education. In some Unitarian churches the sexual education offered is considerably franker and more explicit than most parents would tolerate in a public school. Officials of the Unitarian church have stated a goal of trying to help people with every problem, regardless of its nature. Therefore any problem or question is properly brought up in the church setting. The material used by the Unitarian church is prepared by Dr. Deryck Calderwood and is based on the concept that there is no one established norm of sexual behavior. The teaching departs so far from biblical concepts as to consider them moralistic hangups. It is accepted that young people constantly deal with erotic problems today so they might as well be discussed within an educational framework. The Sunday school course is no "birds and bees" sugar-coated production, but deals with problems of real life, specifically including lovemaking, masturbation, and homosexuality.

Regardless of one's moral code it is clear that sex is a fundamental part of life. There are several purposes that the sex act serves. One of the most obvious is procreation. Speaking on this aspect of sex it is reported that Billy Graham was once questioned by an older lady on his attitude toward sex. He is said to have replied, "Why, ma'am, I'm all for it. Without sex I wouldn't be here and neither would you."

If one accepts that the sex act has other purposes besides procreation, then one opens the door to the universality of sex. Another purpose of sex is simply physical pleasure which may or may not have any association with the emotions ascribed to love.

A third aspect of sex is its use to express love. The importance that is placed upon the sex act has contributed to this. In most people the strongest form of the communication of love one person has for another finds itself in physical, hence sexual, expression.

A fourth and very real purpose of the sex act is its use for psychic fulfillment. An individual's self-image is strongly related to his sexual characteristics. With the emphasis on masculinity within certain societies it is necessary that a man prove to himself his own maleness. Similarly, a woman wishes to feel female. To the extent that these are part of the psychic self-image, the sex act serves as a psychic fulfillment and reassurance of one's maleness, femaleness, or sexuality.

A fifth but very important aspect of the sex act is simple conformity. As indicated in the previous discussion, sexual activity and responses are strongly affected by the social mores of a particular culture. So it is that a woman who may not particularly enjoy sex for a variety of psychic or even physical reasons engages in sexual activity because it is "her marital duty." This is not confined to women. Men, likewise, will perform the sex act because society expects it of them. How the sex act is carried out is usually related to one's concept of what is normal or not normal, regardless of whether these concepts are well founded or not.

The Judeo-Christian concept linking sexuality to evil and sexual abstinence to innocence was responsible for the storm of criticism against Dr. Sigmund Freud when he first presented his views on sexuality and its relationship to the human psyche. The public and his colleagues alike were outraged when he suggested that small children had sexual feelings. The idea that infants were anything besides "sexless angels" so outraged much of the public that many felt Freud's concepts were a matter for the courts. Although Freudian theories are still being debated, it is generally accepted that sexual sensations and identity begin with infancy.

While the baby is still small enough to be bathed by his mother, he begins to learn that the sensation of touching the genitals is pleasurable. With the natural curiosity of childhood, touching, experiencing, and sexual activity begins. The alert young mind seeking information about life and the world about him does not eliminate the sexual sphere, but pursues it as vigorously as any other aspect of his environment. The small child begins to peek at his parents and anyone else when the opportunity provides itself. The boy child compares his anatomy with the girl child and with other boys. Girls, likewise, compare their anatomy with boys and other girls. To function in this vital area of their life they need facts and their childhood curiosity is adequate stimulation to search them out.

Although sexuality in children and young adults has won general acceptance, and for purposes other than procreation, the concept that older individuals are still sexual beings has been somewhat slower to gain acceptance. Many young people are still shocked at the idea that grandma and grandpa would go to bed with each other and do anything besides read the evening paper or watch TV. Sexual interest begins early and remains to the very end of the life span. This is clearly pointed out by the many letters from older people which I have received. Many older women remain products of the Victorian era, but still others frankly describe their sexual drive even though they are seventy years of age or older and have long since passed their menopausal period. Many men retain sexual interest into their nineties. The despair of many older men over the problem of impotence exemplifies clearly that even after the flesh is no longer able, the mind is still hopeful.

There are many psychiatrists who believe that a large number of other aspects of living are indirectly related to fundamental sex drives and sexual behavior, aside from direct sexual acts and desires. The woman's interest in her kitchen and her home is described as a "nesting" drive of femininity. Different forms of daily activity are described as

10

expressing one's masculinity or femininity. The persistent football enthusiast and spectator sports addict is said to gain expression of his sexual drive through his sport. These views serve to point out the philosophy held by some that even the most remote aspects of our living habits are in essence expressions of our sexuality.

Despite all that has been learned and presented on sexual matters, the experience of receiving thousands of letters from individuals concerning sexual problems adds a new dimension to human sexuality. Such letters raise real questions as opposed to theoretical considerations. It is difficult to find information on the problem posed by many women who write to ask about their husbands' preference for masturbation rather than intercourse. There is the wife who expresses her concern over the possibility that she may get cancer because her husband has cancer of the prostate gland. The letters have emphasized to me the very frequent concern of middle-aged women about pregnancy. Many of these women want to know when they can enjoy sexual activity without taking the usual precautions for birth control. They often ask if they can still get pregnant after their menstrual periods have ceased. Through their letters, individuals have defined the real areas of concern that most people experience in their active sex lives today.

The stories that people have told me, recounting the problems of their own life, coupled with the history of sex through time and in different civilizations reveals quite clearly that sex begins and ends with life, and no matter how it is altered through cultural influences and social pressures, it must be accepted that sex is, always was, and ever shall be. It remains for us to understand more completely the nature of our own sexuality.

How one chooses to conduct his own sex life is really a very personal matter of primary concern to the individual and his or her sexual partner. What is right or wrong depends to a large extent upon whether it is harmful or not harmful to the individual or any other being. Not infrequently something is considered harmful only because it conflicts with our preconceived notions, which really reflect our ignorance.

The problems of sex are not solved by ignorance. Dr. Allen Gregg, who introduced Dr. Kinsey's book, *Human Sexuality in the Male,* expressed this concept well, stating: "Insofar as man seeks to know himself and face his whole nature, he has become free from bewildered fear, despondent shame, or arrant hypocrisy." Understanding one's sexuality, or being aware that what one may assume to be a unique problem is indeed commonplace, serves to help one develop a better base of information from which to decide how best to conduct one's life. Sweeping away misconceptions and replacing them with knowledge is fundamental to progress and mental health. In the words of one of the great teachers, "the truth shall make you free."

II

Doing What Comes Naturally

DOING WHAT COMES NATURALLY may conflict with the codes of our society. As moral standards change, some conflicts are resolved while others are aggravated.

VIRGINITY

High on the list of concerns is the persistent question about virginity. Sexual freedom has not totally erased the value set on arriving at the marital bed in a virginal state. Most letters I receive expressing anxiety about virginity are from girls. There is an occasional young man who is being pressured toward marriage by a girl who claims to be pregnant even though, according to the young man, they have never actually engaged in sexual intercourse. This situation raises the question of defining a virgin.

In its broadest definition a virgin may simply be "an unmarried woman." In its strictest definition it could mean a person who had no form of physical contact with members of the opposite sex, or, in fact, sexual experience of any type. The question remains, how chaste do you have to be to be a virgin. American society commonly uses the term to indicate that the girl's hymen membrane at the outlet of the vagina is still intact, the physical proof that the maiden has not been "sexually violated." The notion that a girl must have an intact hymen on her wedding night is closely akin to a tribal custom when villagers waited outside the nuptial quarters until a bloody cloth was tossed out of the bridal window as proof of the girl's chastity.

The hymen membrane can be destroyed by means other than sexual intercourse. When it is rigid, unmovable, or is a significant mechanical block to sexual activity it should be removed prior to beginning sexual activity.

Dear Dr. Lamb—I am about to be married in a couple of months and I'm a nervous wreck. When I was younger I had relations with someone I loved very much, so therefore I am no longer a virgin. Could you tell me if my husband will be able to tell on my wedding night whether or not I am a virgin? If so, is there any explanation I can use? I am terribly upset and don't want anything to spoil my marriage. How do other girls explain this?

Comment—It is usually much better if such problems are resolved before marriage rather than allowing them to become confrontations on the wedding night. Marriage does not thrive well when individuals keep important secrets from each other, particularly if the secret causes extreme anxiety in either person. A girl who is seriously worried about what her future mate will think of her previous sexual activity would be well advised to discuss this area with her prospective husband and resolve these conflicts before the actual ceremony. The intelligent, well-adjusted person usually marries another individual for what they are rather than what they were, and for what they hope they will do and how they will behave in the future rather than what they have done in the past.

All girls planning to be married should have a careful premarital examination. Many virgins are not physiologically equipped for the sex act and are more apt to start off a happy married life if potential problems are prevented in advance. This includes being examined to be certain that the vaginal canal will be prepared for sexual intercourse. If the hymen membrane is tough or rigid, a premarital incision or removal of the hymen is necessary. For those who feel that they absolutely must have an explanation for being prepared for an active sexual life, the obvious and very often the proper explanation is that their physician has removed the mechanical obstruction so that sexual activity can be a pleasure instead of a painful and disappointing experience.

Writing on this problem, Dr. Robert Dickinson, a specialist in obstetrics and gynecology and author of *Human Sex Anatomy,* instructs young women in how to prepare themselves for their wedding night. He points out that the vagina of a girl who has not used a douche nozzle or been examined or handled in any way is so small that the average forefinger is passed with difficulty if at all. As the finger is inserted it encounters a sensitive edge (the hymen) which can gradually be stretched and desensitized. Dr. Dickinson, like many other physicians, instructs such a girl in procedures to enlarge the vaginal opening. She begins with a well-lubricated fingertip and gently inserts it. She progresses to two fingers, and then three fingers, inserting them as far as she can reach. This is done daily or twice a day for ten to fourteen days before the wedding.

If a very tight vagina is not prepared it cannot admit an erect penis without difficulty and pain. This can lead to a lifetime of sexual maladjustment and unhappiness for both mates, a high price to pay for being able to prove the girl has been untouched by human hands or anything else.

This problem can also be avoided by a gradual buildup to coitus between a couple over a period of days if the girl is not experienced. This approach with gradual penetration will allow the vaginal vault to slowly dilate and be receptive to sex. Many men, not appreciating this problem, charge on with disastrous results for the launching of the girl's active sex life.

In a woman who has been properly prepared, discomfort will be slight, if it occurs at all. The worst that will happen is a couple of nicks or notches, usually less than a quarter of an inch deep, and there should be no more than a drop or two of blood, or none at all.

Dear Dr. Lamb—I would like to know if a nineteen- or twenty-year-old girl is a virgin if she has had sexual intercourse between the ages of four and nine. She didn't start her periods until about the age of fifteen.

Comment—This letter is an indication of the early sexual activity that frequently occurs in children. While virginity is a matter of definition, penetration of the vagina at any age can potentially rupture the hymen membrane. The time of onset of menstrual flow in relation to previous sexual activity has nothing to do with the anatomical aspects of virginity. Incidentally, for the normal discharge of the menstrual blood flow it is necessary that the hymen membrane be partially perforated. In rare instances where no perforation is present the menstrual flow will be occluded and the hymen will have to be incised for normal menses to occur.

It should be added that any girl who has not been sexually active from ages nine to fifteen is likely to have a small, tight vaginal vault, whether or not a hymen membrane is present.

Dear Dr. Lamb—I am twenty-two. My boyfriend (we're engaged) is twenty-six and I want to wait until we are married before we actually do sexual intercourse. I am still a virgin. I know that, but we have done it halfway, but not all the way. Please, I'm worried sick, can you be a virgin and still be pregnant?

Comment—Whether or not a virgin can be pregnant is entirely dependent upon one's definition of virginity. Certainly a girl cannot be pregnant if there has been no form of sexual play. Sexual activity must have gone far enough that the penis discharged some semen near or at the opening of the vaginal orifice.

The sperm are motile and if they are placed at the opening of the vagina, it is possible that they could pass through the vagina into the uterus to the tube to meet a waiting ovum, with pregnancy resulting. This could all occur with the hymen being relatively intact. Obviously, there must be an opening in the hymen if the sperm is to pass from the vagina into the uterus. This opening, though, could be the normal one expected for the passage of the menstrual blood flow.

It should be pointed out that the initial drops of semen contain the largest number of sperm cells. One small drop in the right location at the right time is sufficient to induce pregnancy. Sexual activity or "heavy petting" that causes the male to discharge at the vaginal opening even without full penetration has the potential of inducing a surprise pregnancy.

Dear Dr. Lamb—I am eighteen years of age and am planning to be married next month. My fiancé has just returned from Vietnam two weeks ago and I haven't had the courage to confess to him that I engaged in sexual intercourse three times while he was away. The last time was four months ago. Will my fiancé be able to sense my lack of virginity? Is there any way I could prevent him from finding out? I was told that operations are being performed which could conceal this fact. Is this true? If so, could you explain the operation and the cost.

Comment—This letter suggests that the girl has not had sexual relations with her fiancé. Otherwise there would be no question about whether she is a virgin or not. There are operations for placing an artificial hymen in the vagina. However these are not routinely done and it would be very difficult for most people to find a physician who would be willing to do this procedure. For the girl who feels her only solution to this difficult problem is deception, her best approach is through the premarital examination so that her future husband will not expect her to have a tight vagina or a hymen membrane that needs to be ruptured.

It might be added that the presence of a hymen membrane itself is not conclusive evidence that a girl has not participated in sexual intercourse. The hymen membrane, after all, is merely a thin stretched piece of tissue at the vaginal opening. If it stretches sufficiently, it is possible for the penis to penetrate under the edge of the hymen membrane without actually tearing or ripping it. This, however, is relatively unusual.

17

Dear Dr. Lamb—This may sound like a dumb question but please answer. If a female and male have clothes on, could the female possibly get pregnant? This worries me terribly.

Comment—This is not the dumb question that the girl thinks it is. It depends on what is meant by clothed. If semen seeps through the clothing to the vaginal orifice, there is of course the possibility of pregnancy. It would seem unlikely, though, that semen would reach this location unless at least the male penis was next to the underwear of the girl. Girls have gotten pregnant without removing their underwear.

SEX FREQUENCY

There is a great deal of concern about how frequently sexual relations should take place. Many letters indicate that there is often a mismatch between the sexual desires of the man and the woman. Almost all the letters on this problem come from women, since men do not write complaining that their wives do not like to have sex, or that their wives want sex more often than they do. Women who do not desire to have sex frequently often are classified as "frigid" and these problems are discussed in the chapter on female sexual dysfunction. Many people seem to think that there is a magic number and any number more or less frequent is abnormal. The concern about that aspect of the problem of frequency is a good example of sexual conformity by the numbers.

Dear Dr. Lamb—I have been married for five years and my question is what are the average times for a couple to have relations. I still feel like having relations every other day, but sometimes my husband doesn't ask for it for maybe a whole week. He used to be a very virile man, wanting love two or three times a night. I am always fixed up and wear perfume and pretty nightgowns, but they seem to do absolutely nothing. If I were sloppy or dirty I could understand. I've tried sitting down and talking it over and I've come right out and asked him why he doesn't want to make love as often any more and one time he said he just wasn't in the mood and another time he just laughed it off and wouldn't answer me.

He swears he has no one else and I believe him. Is it really normal for a man married only five years and in his twenties to be this disinterested in sex?

I know I'm still attractive because other men are always admiring me. If I only knew why this was so, maybe I could solve the problem but not knowing is quite distressing. I know he's not impotent because I've seen him aroused to the fullest in bed but he never turns to me for fulfillment. He just waits for it to subside and goes about his business for the day. I would like to get our marriage back to a mutually satisfactory sex life. I don't believe I'm oversexed for this, but I have noticed that as I get older I grow more sexually stimulated compared to my teen years. I am in my twenties and it feels good to have a satisfactory sex life with my husband. I am not one of those women who are always tired and refuse their husbands for many stupid reasons. I would never cheat on my husband as it is against all my beliefs, religious, moral, and otherwise. I need help about my dilemma.

Comment—On the surface this appears to be a simple problem of mismatch in desire. It is not unusual to desire sexual intercourse only once a week. The simple truth is that there are different levels of sexual desire in both the male and female. A woman may be entirely satisfied to have sex only once a week or she may desire it more frequently, as in this case. The same is true of a man. Sexual harmony in a marriage is most often achieved when both partners have about the same frequency of desire.

Of course, sexual desire is markedly affected by many other factors. It's interesting to note that the husband in this case was accustomed to having sex regularly two to three times a night at the beginning of their married sex life. No doubt this is the period of the greatest emotional, romantic love. Mental and emotional factors are powerful influences on the frequency of sexual desire. When a person meets another individual who strongly stimulates him sexually, the entire sexual system is literally turned on. This includes the stimulation of the endocrine glands. A good example of this is the influence on the beard growth of the man. It has been demonstrated that when a man is in isolation away from sexual opportunity, the growth of his beard slows markedly. Just before he returns from isolation to sexual opportunity his beard begins to grow rapidly and continues to do so for the first two to three days of sexual activity. After this, the beard growth begins to slow. These and numerous other examples indicate the influence of the psyche over the hormone and sexual system. The two are really in balance. The hormones will influence the psyche, and the psyche will influence the hormones.

The best solution to the problems of mismatch in frequency is an understanding by both individuals that there may normally be different levels of sexual desire. This helps to remove the distrust and suspicion that sometimes creeps into these situations.

Within the marriage framework it is usually expected that both parties will make an effort to please each other and fill each other's needs. This ideal situation cannot always be obtained, however, and it serves little purpose to beg, cajole, nag, or otherwise introduce unpleasant emotional experiences into an already overly sensitive environment. The wife who does everything that she can to be a loving wife and support her husband's ego is more apt to have a sexy husband. There is still a place for salesmanship and courtship regarding sexual matters within the marriage, and this applies to both partners. It usually accomplishes much more than complaining.

Dear Dr. Lamb—My husband and I fight constantly as he thinks you must have sex three or four times a week. He would rather have sex than eat. I am of the opinion that there's more to life than that. I am not against sex, but twice a week is more than enough. It would be different if he enjoyed it, but he seems to force himself. He is forty-three, and I am thirty-six. We have no children as I had to have surgery a few years ago and can't have them. The problem is he keeps telling me there is something wrong with me, and I am beginning to get a complex thinking he may be right. Is there something wrong with me, or is he oversexed?

Comment—There is really nothing wrong with either one of these people. They just exemplify the difference in the level of desire for intercourse. Neither two times nor four times a week is particularly unusual, nor is once every two weeks or seven times a week. The best thing to do about the numbers game is to forget it and enjoy sexual relations without keeping score.

Dear Dr. Lamb—Is it good for a male or a female to have intercourse every night? Also, is it the best idea for a fellow to lie on his wife with all his weight?

Comment—Every night is not unusual for some couples, and if both individuals are in good health with no medical problems, there is no reason it should cause any difficulties.

Usually the wife enjoys sexual relations more if she is comfortable. If her husband places too much weight on her and she is uncomfortable, she should tell him so. It is absolutely amazing how two individuals living close enough together to have regular sexual activities, in this instance apparently every night, have difficulty in telling each other what they like and do not like. After all, sexual expression is an extremely important aspect of life and one that should be discussed.

Dear Dr. Lamb—I am really getting desperate and I can't bring myself to talk to my doctor about it, because it would embarrass me and I'm afraid he'll think I'm whacky. I'm in my early forties and my husband is in his early fifties. We've been married over twenty years and up until the last few months we've had a normal sex life. Now I seem to want sex more often than he does. He only wants it about once a week. I want it two or three times a week. Is that too much?

He says he loves me, but he doesn't show it, but he is a good provider and a good father. I'd like to have fewer material things and a little more love. I've got my weight down and know that I'm attractive. Do you think my husband has been unfaithful? I feel sometimes that maybe this is it. I need and must be loved or I feel I will do something desperate like finding another man. I have no one in mind and was raised in a nice home and never went to bars or anything like that. I feel that this is why women and men drift apart and do wrong, because their mate does not understand them. My husband thinks I'm oversexed and I say I'm not. I'm just human and he should be glad I'm that way instead of being cold. Please advise me before it's too late.

Comment—A woman's sexual desire often increases in her middle years. This is true even after the menopause. There are many reasons for this. After the menopause some women feel liberated from the fears of pregnancy. Another important factor is the identity with youth. A woman who is sexually active feels she is still young, and this can be important to a woman who is actually getting older.

The man this writer describes also seems normal. Men do tend to have a decrease in their level of sexual desire as they get older. It would not be uncommon for a man in his early fifties to want sexual activity only about once a week. This, of course, varies widely with the individual concerned. Sometimes when real difficulties arise because of different levels of desire, it is well for the couple to discuss the problem with a qualified marriage counselor. Discussing the problem in the presence of a third party often clears the air. This woman needs reassurance that her husband's sexual desire is not abnormal and is not an indication that he is unfaithful.

22

Dear Dr. Lamb—My husband is undersexed. Is there anything he can take to increase his sex appetite? I mean medicine, not sex potions of some sort. He's twenty-nine and we've been married four years. He is completely satisfied to have relations only three times a month or less. He was like this when we had been married only one and a half or two years. This is frustrating, humiliating, and heartbreaking to a wife. I am reasonably attractive and keep myself clean so that isn't the problem. Many women have this problem but feel too ashamed to discuss it. If there is a medicine a man can take, is it harmful in any way? I know my husband isn't stepping out and he isn't gay either.

Comment—This is just another example of mismatch in sexual appetite. Unless a young man truly has a medical problem (which is quite rare), there are no medicines that are useful for this purpose and some which might be used could actually be harmful. Administration of male hormone, for example, for a man who has a normal amount of hormone to begin with may actually depress the normal function of the testicles in producing sperm.

Dear Dr. Lamb—My husband and I have been married eight years and are in our latter twenties. Most of our married life has been lived with little or no sex. What physiological effects could develop in my husband and myself if no mutual love-sex relationship can be developed?

Comment—Although sex is very important in marriage, it is only one of the many aspects of such a complicated relationship. Many people do live apparently happy lives with minimal sexual activity. There are also records of individuals who have been married for many years without ever having consummated the marriage, although it is difficult to understand how such a situation could be happy or physiologically satisfying. If there is little or no "love-sex relationship" merely by mutual desire and it is not caused by some underlying medical problem, there is no reason that it should

23

cause any biological disturbance.

Dear Dr. Lamb—I have been married seven years and our sex life lasted only six months. My husband is diabetic. Whenever I made any remark he would say he had a backache or some other cute excuse, so I finally said I wanted a baby. Then two years later we had a baby. Right then, sex died. I went on thinking it was illness, so I suffered in silence. Then I discovered he was having an affair. I accused him of this, which ended up in a row.

To make a long story short, I began to neglect his clothes and meals until he complained I wasn't looking after him properly, so I told him why and this resulted in another big row. So he got cross and told me the truth. The reason was he didn't find me as physically attractive as he thought I would be. Well, that was worse than if he had put a knife through my heart. I never hated anyone so much before. Then he was sorry for having told me this. He said he loved me and sex is not the only reason for staying together.

I think we made our mistake in the beginning because we were both too shy. He thought I knew all about sex and that's where he made his mistake. My mother used to say it was the husband's duty to teach his wife sex. Now I don't know what to do. I am so unhappy and ashamed of myself and afraid to be sexual. My husband says now that we must try again, but I don't know what to do. Have you any suggestions to help us?

Comment—This is the type of problem that really needs a marriage counselor. On the surface, the woman's letter would seem to indicate that both parties would like to have a satisfactory marriage with a satisfactory sexual life. Her letter also suggests that they began having difficulty at the onset of their marriage because of sexual ignorance. This isn't particularly unusual. There are probably as many difficulties in marriage caused by sexual ignorance as there are

24

by psychological factors. This is one of the reasons that healthy sex education is important for a healthy normal life.

Dear Dr. Lamb—I have a question I wish you would answer. This is about to destroy our marriage. My husband was overseas for a year. When he came home on leave, he wouldn't make love to me. Since he has been home three months, he still won't make love to me. I've asked him why and he says he doesn't know why. I try to touch him and he won't let me. He's only thirty-nine and I know this couldn't be normal. Is there anywhere we could get help?

Comment—While there are individual differences in the level of sexual desire, a total absence of desire is not normal. It is true that a person may not particularly desire to engage in sexual activity with another specific person. In this instance the husband may not wish to have sex with his wife even though he may still have a normal sex drive. If that were the case, it would be based on their interpersonal relationship which would need exploring. If the husband's behavior represents a total lack of interest in sex, he deserves psychiatric help. Ideally the husband should see his family physician, who no doubt would give him a relatively complete medical examination to rule out any medical problems, and he should ask his doctor to refer him to a psychiatrist for professional counseling. An absence of sexual interest may not necessarily indicate an important sexual problem and it may even be related to an emotional depression which in this instance might be related to the man's recently terminated military service.

Dear Dr. Lamb—I read your column about the fifty-two-year-old woman who didn't intend to give up sex at her age. I have news for her. I have been married eighteen years and can count on my fingers how many times I enjoyed my sex act with my husband. He never cared about sex. He is an ardent sportsman and I mean ardent. If by any chance I mention the sex act and why he married me, to torture me or what, he gets furious. I can't discuss anything about sex with him. It has made me very nervous and caused me to cry many times, but now at forty-six years of age it doesn't bother me that much.

I would never have lived all of these years with him but somehow accidentally we had two children and to keep peace I keep quiet. Could you tell me if he is hiding anything? Are there men who can't perform the act or what? I hear some of my friends say "My husband is always bothering me." What is the solution to such a predicament?

Comment—If the problem is as bad as the letter suggests the only real solution is professional counseling for both parties. This letter illustrates one point. "Ardent sportsmen" and "he-men" are not necessarily athletic or sporty in the bedroom. Sometimes these "masculine activities" cover a man's insecurity in the sexual sphere. Taunting, cajoling, and confrontation will not help build up his confidence but will merely make matters worse. Sexual performance is often a matter of confidence. Repeated success is a powerful sexual stimulus.

INTERCOURSE AND PREGNANCY

Many women are concerned about the effects of intercourse on their pregnancy. This is particularly true if the woman has previously lost a child.

Dear Dr. Lamb—About two years ago I gave birth to a baby girl who had died twelve hours before delivery. The doctor said that it was just one of those things and that the placenta had given way. Now I am expecting another baby and I am scared that the same thing will happen again. Could intercourse be wrong?

Dear Dr. Lamb—I am expecting my first child and would like to know if it is dangerous or if there is any harm

26

in having intercourse while being pregnant. In a couple of weeks I'll be eight months along and I'm worried about what will happen if I continue to have intercourse. Is it good or bad? Please explain why or why not.

Dear Dr. Lamb—I am twenty years old and am expecting my first baby. When I first realized I was pregnant I began having a lot of trouble with bleeding and dizziness. However, I have been under a doctor's care and have not had any trouble for the past two months. I'm carrying the baby very low and the lower muscles hurt so bad that I have to limp around.

My husband is in the army and is stationed in Japan and I'm going to join him this month. I can't help but wonder if the bleeding I had before was caused by intercourse we had one night. Perhaps it wasn't, but do you think it would be very wise for us to have intercourse when I get there?

I am concerned from the sound of his last two letters since he is looking forward to sex much too eagerly. We have been married eight months and separated three months, and I know he's very eager for sex. He said he probably wouldn't do much sleeping for a few nights. I know this is all very personal but I must talk to someone about it. I love my baby and don't want to take chances.

Comment—Unless there are some unusual difficulties with the pregnancy, there are usually no contraindications to having sexual relations during the first eight months. Many obstetricians will permit it until four weeks before delivery. It is a good idea to ask the obstetrician what his wishes are in this regard.

If a woman is threatened with miscarriage, as evidenced by bleeding and cramping, it is certainly unwise to engage in any form of physical activity, and such a woman should be under a doctor's care. Usually he will restrict her activity and probably ask her to stay in bed. If the event passes and the pregnancy proceeds in a normal fashion, there is no reason that sexual activity should be curtailed. The girl who is going to see her army husband must have been pregnant for at least four months, since they have been separated for three. This should mean that she is past the early phase of pregnancy when threatened miscarriages are more likely, and it should mean she would be in a period when sexual relations would not pose any real threat to the pregnancy. The usual reasons for curtailing sexual intercourse immediately before delivery are merely to minimize the likelihood of introducing any bacteria into the vaginal canal just before the delivery and further to minimize the possibility of early rupture of the fetal membranes. Even this is relatively unlikely.

Recent studies show that when a woman has an orgasm it causes uterine contractions. This can induce early labor or in the early months of pregnancy contribute to miscarriage. This is equally true if the orgasm occurs by any means besides sexual intercourse. If intercourse occurs without an orgasm this will not happen. Thus, the man can have an orgasm and as long as the woman doesn't, uterine contractions won't be stimulated. Although there are many other causes, uterine contractions can be a factor in premature separation of the placenta, which is what the first lady described as a cause for her baby's death. This is more apt to occur close to the time of delivery and is a good reason why the woman should avoid having an orgasm during the final month of pregnancy.

There is one other danger from sex during pregnancy. If during oral-genital relations, the man forces air into the vagina it can be absorbed by the many blood vessels in the pregnant uterus and the air bubble can get in the mother's circulation and even cause death.

STRANGE NYMPHO

Dear Dr. Lamb—I won't go through any mumbo-jumbo.

I'll come right to the point. I think I'm a nymphomaniac. I know that it's normal to have "the urge" but to be thinking about it all day and even dreaming about it gets very troublesome. The bad thing about it is I'm only fifteen years old. I'm very mature for my age but it doesn't alter the fact that I think my teen-age sex drive is a lot stronger than usual. I'm still a virgin, unlike almost everyone else I know.

I can't talk to anyone, my parents or counselors, because I'd be awfully embarrassed, and even my sister who is the closest person to me doesn't have the slightest idea. I can't go to a psychiatrist because I don't have the money. Please help me.

Comment—Whoever heard of a nymphomaniac who was a virgin? It's perfectly normal for a teen-ager to have frequent and almost constant thoughts about sex. These are often the years when the sex drive is the strongest. Because people seem to think they're unusual, it's not too uncommon for them to bottle up their problems and not discuss them with anyone else. Usually what they discuss with other people is fanciful and not the areas of real concern. It does help to talk about one's feelings and no doubt this girl would have considerable relief about her problems if she could bring herself to discuss her feelings and reactions with someone that she cared a great deal about, for example. her sister. She might be surprised to find out that even her sister experiences strong sexual feelings.

WET DREAMS

There appears to be widespread misinterpretation about the significance of nocturnal emissions, or "wet dreams." They can be a source of anxiety when they are not understood.

Dear Dr. Lamb—About once or twice a week I dream at night that I am seducing a girl and when I wake up I have a discharge on my underwear. Can you tell me what this means? I was wondering if this could be a sign of VD.

Dear Dr. Lamb—Would you please comment on nocturnal emissions or wet dreams. What would cause a thirty-six-year-old married man to have frequent wet dreams? I am anxious to know what some of the causes might be and also if there is any preventative. Obviously, something is amiss somewhere along the line and I'd appreciate any information or advice you might be able to give.

Comment—A nocturnal emission is certainly not an indication of venereal disease. It is a normal event and the common term, wet dream, is very appropriate. Study of sleep and dreaming activity in recent years has demonstrated that dreams can be identified by rapid eye movement (REM) seen on the record of the brain's electrical activity. The REM occurs periodically during the night in normal people. In men this is the time when a nocturnal erection may occur. The erection is totally out of control of the conscious mind of the person. These may occur several times during the night associated with erotic dreams. In the course of the dream full sexual stimulation with actual discharge can occur. This is particularly apt to occur in men who have a very strong sex drive and do not have an opportunity for its fulfillment. Hence, it's common in young boys when they are at the height of their sexual stimulation and are often limited in their sexual opportunity. However, it is not abnormal for it to occur in anyone, whether young, old, single, or married. Kinsey and his co-workers reported that nocturnal orgasms during sleep were acknowledged by 37 percent of women surveyed and at least 80 percent of the men.

It must be remembered that just because a man is married doesn't mean that he has turned off all sources of sexual stimulation other than his wife. He is still exposed to the erotic stimulation of normal living and regardless of how vir-

30

tuous he is, he has relatively little control over his dream life. Then, of course, his erotic dreams may involve his wife. In any case, it is not a matter to be concerned about as long as the other aspects of sexual life are satisfactory. The same applies to sexual dreams for women.

VAGINAL OR CLITORAL ORGASM

For years, great controversy raged about the relative importance of vaginal or clitoral orgasms in women. No doubt some of these misconceptions will be a long time in dying.

Dear Dr. Lamb—Do you agree with the opinion that women should not expect vaginal orgasm because it doesn't exist? Would you consider one who does have such an orgasm to have a physical or emotional problem?

Comment—One of the important achievements of the Masters and Johnson research was to demonstrate objectively what a female orgasm is. Their studies should have laid to rest once and for all the controversies surrounding vaginal or clitoral orgasms. Expressed in the terminology of Gertrude Stein, an orgasm is an orgasm is an orgasm. When a female experiences an orgasm, it is a total response. It affects the skin color of the female genitalia and involves the total sexual apparatus—even the female breasts undergo changes. This relatively total response is not limited to either the clitoris or the vagina. It is also interesting to note that those women who've had the clitoris removed can still experience a complete, effective orgasm. There is no such thing as maturity or immaturity associated with having either a clitoral or vaginal orgasm. A woman may be stimulated to orgasm through a variety of mechanisms including stimulation of the clitoris or stimulation of the lips or labia of the vagina, but the actual orgasm itself is a total response. A woman who thinks she's having a vaginal orgasm is really having "an orgasm."

THE FERTILE PERIOD

Despite all the available sexual information, it's surprising how many people have no clear concept of when a woman is most likely to get pregnant. There is widespread misunderstanding or lack of knowledge about the normal menstrual cycle.

Dear Dr. Lamb—My husband and I don't want any kids as of now. I have heard from friends that there is a certain time when you can have sex and not get pregnant. Is this so? If so, when is the time?

Dear Dr. Lamb—Please answer this question. What is the usual time for a woman to get pregnant? I have heard so many things I don't know which is right. None seem to work for me.

Comment—Although there is great variability in different people and even in the same woman between cycles, the classic concept is that a woman is most fertile at the midpoint between periods. Specifically, this is fourteen days before the onset of menstruation. To allow for variability, the period between the twelfth and sixteenth days between the menstrual cycle is considered the most fertile time for a regular woman with a twenty-eight-day cycle.

The first day of blood flow or menstruation is called day one. Menstruation is the dismantling or sloughing off of the lining of the womb if pregnancy does not occur. The sloughing literally is the result of a decrease in the amount of female hormones that have been generated to prepare for pregnancy. Immediately after the lining is sloughed off, the uterus begins preparation for another attempt at pregnancy. While the new ovum (egg) is ripening for the intended pregnancy, female hormone (estrogen) pours out and stimulates the formation of a new lining of the womb.

At about the fourteenth day, the blisterlike formation in the ovary that encloses the egg actually ruptures, releasing the ovum. The ovum passes into the open mouth of the tube and starts down the horn or the tube toward the uterus. While it's in the tube, if it meets a live sperm cell and the two join, pregnancy occurs. Even if this doesn't happen, preparation for pregnancy continues with the further development of the lining of the womb. Fourteen days after the ovum has been released into the tube, if it wasn't impregnated, menstruation will start. Thus you can judge by hindsight when a woman was susceptible to pregnancy. The problems occur when a woman isn't regular. Hindsight is sometimes too late if one wants to prevent a pregnancy by knowing when ovulation occurred.

Dear Dr. Lamb—Is it possible for conception to occur immediately after a menstrual period or right before it? Urgent!

Comment—Yes. In a woman who is not regular, another ovum may be prepared and released early. If a pregnancy didn't occur, the next period would also be early. It is not so easy to get pregnant immediately preceding a menstrual period and these are usually considered fairly safe days for sexual activity without causing pregnancy. The problem is that one doesn't always know when the next menstrual period will be. If the woman is late in ovulating, menstruation occurs later, much to the concern of both parties.

Dear Dr. Lamb—Is it possible to have intercourse eight days before a woman's period and have her in a family way? How long does it take the sperm to catch a woman and make her pregnant?

Comment—Although classically a woman menstruates fourteen days after she ovulates, there are frequent variations. Some women ovulate without menstruating at all, or the flow may be so minimal or scanty that it will not be noticed. Then there are such things as spotting or bleeding from factors other than the regular menstrual period. Some women bleed at the midpoint in their menstrual period at the actual time of ovulation, which confuses the issue even more. These variations make it impossible to be dogmatic about the relationship of pregnancy to menstrual periods.

The sperm usually live about forty-eight hours. The ovum from the woman, however, only lives about six or eight hours. If a woman has had intercourse the day before she ovulates, then she may have live sperm in her tubes just waiting for the ovum.

Dear Dr. Lamb—Does ovulation occur during pregnancy?
Comment—No. Ovulation is actually stimulated by hormones that come from the small pituitary gland resting underneath the brain. Hormones formed by the ovaries in the early part of pregnancy and by the placenta in the latter part of pregnancy block the release of the hormone from the pituitary gland that stimulates ovulation. This, by the way, is how birth control pills work. They use female hormones that block the pituitary gland from causing ovulation.

Dear Dr. Lamb—Is it possible and what are the chances of becoming pregnant during the monthly period?
Comment—Theoretically, it's possible. In some animals, incidentally, sexual intercourse stimulates ovulation. It is relatively unlikely, however, for a woman to be ovulating during the menstrual period.

Dear Dr. Lamb—I have had eight children with my first marriage. Then I had an operation so I couldn't have any more. I remarried and had an operation so that I could have children again. Eight years passed and the last six years I didn't even have a period. Now my doctor tells me I am five months pregnant. How can I get pregnant if I didn't have a period for six years? A pregnancy test was also made and it was positive. I look it and feel it and am in wonderful health and happy about the whole thing. So is my husband. We thank God each night for my being pregnant again. Can you really get pregnant if you haven't had a period?

Comment—This is a happy outcome to correction of an earlier sterilization operation. Having a period and getting pregnant are two different things. Whenever the ovum is fertilized, a woman is pregnant. Menstruation is merely the shedding of the lining of the womb. It's not rare for women to ovulate and not menstruate. Failure to realize this has caused some women to assume that they can't get pregnant because they're not menstruating.

Dear Dr. Lamb—I have a problem. I am eighteen years old and have a ten-month-old girl. Now I am going to have another child and when I was one or two months along I had two or three relationships with another guy. Do you think the baby will look like him, and if he said he couldn't have any kids and you had a relationship with him and left the sperm in the body until the next morning, could you still have his baby? I love him very much.

Do you think I am too young to have my tubes tied? Please tell me what to do. I am so mixed up.

Comment—It's not clear from her letter whether this girl is married or not. In any case, if she's pregnant, having relations with another man after the pregnancy has already occurred won't influence the characteristics of the expected child, and the second man can't be the father.

Unless there is some important medical reason for it, an eighteen-year-old girl should not have her tubes tied. The procedure is often irreversible, and there are a lot of things that happen in a person's life after their first eighteen years.

MEN'S CYCLE

Dear Dr. Lamb—As a married woman with an eighteen-month-old baby, the question I am about to ask may seem absurd to say the least. I've had no classroom sex education. I have had to learn through wives tales, "girl talk," and my husband (who knew less than I did). However, my question is this. I know that there are fertile and unfertile days for women. Are there fertile and unfertile days for men? Are there certain emotional qualities that can lower the sperm count, or make the sperm less active? When intercourse is repeated and a second ejaculation occurs, are the sperm cells weaker then or simply less in number, which in turn would reduce the possibility of conceiving?

Comment—Men don't have sperm cycles in the same way that women have ovulatory cycles. Sperm cells are constantly being generated in the body of the testicle and then ripening to maturity in the coiled tube lying next to the body of the testicle. (Incidentally, sperm are not stored in the prostate or the seminal vessicle pouches of the male.) The largest number of sperm cells are discharged in the first few drops of the semen. The rest of the seminal fluid is made up of secretions from the prostate gland and other parts of the man's reproductive system. You can't make a blanket guarantee that there will be fewer sperm cells in the second ejaculation, but this is a good probability. As a general guideline, most doctors who are doing fertility studies on men ask them not to have sexual activity for three or sometimes five days before a sample is obtained for study. This implies that abstinence from sexual activity for three days would cause a maximum amount of sperm cells to be present in the sample.

There are many factors which influence the number of sperm cells, including the overall health of the man. These are discussed further in the questions concerning male fertility.

CALCULATING PREGNANCY DATE

Dear Dr. Lamb—Can a woman become pregnant two weeks after her last sexual intercourse with a man, and can a doctor be more than a week off in calculating the time of the pregnancy?

Comment—The sperm cells only live about forty-eight hours. However, it's not so easy to determine when a woman has ovulated and when she actually got pregnant or will deliver. If doctors could tell exactly when a woman got pregnant, they'd be a lot more accurate in determining when a woman is going to deliver, although there are other factors involved. I would say it's entirely possible for a physician to misjudge when a woman became pregnant, by at least two to three weeks in some cases.

SIGNS OF PREGNANCY

Dear Dr. Lamb—I am a married girl, aged seventeen, and I think I am pregnant, but I don't know any signs of pregnancy because I've never had a baby before. The only thing that makes me think I am is that my breasts are very sore, and I haven't had a period this month. But you can't always tell whether you are pregnant by your menstrual periods, I guess. I have been having menstrual periods only every two or three months lately. Could you please tell me some signs of pregnancy.

Also, is it possible for a woman to not miss a monthly period and still be pregnant?

Comment—The early diagnosis of pregnancy isn't so easy unless one uses laboratory tests. Even though it is not always a reliable sign, missing a regular menstrual period is highly suggestive of pregnancy. In many instances it is the first symptom which the woman herself notes. This early in the pregnancy even a physical examination by a doctor may not give a ready answer to the question. A little later in the pregnancy, of course, there are changes in the female genitalia, some of which are not conclusive but are strongly suggestive on physical examination. Also, the doctor can feel the early enlargement of the pregnant uterus. Then, of course, the breasts do begin to enlarge under the influence of increased amounts of female hormones produced during the pregnancy. A little later some women develop pigmented spots on their face which has been called the "mask of pregnancy." Many women are said to be at their most beautiful during their first pregnancy. For this reason, many artists have chosen to paint a woman's portrait during her first pregnancy when she is "in full bloom."

A woman can also be pregnant even though she has menstrual periods. Thus, having a period cannot be used as a definite sign that a woman is not pregnant. On rare occasions a woman may have menstrual periods for quite some time after she is actually pregnant. Then there is the problem of confusing spotting, which sometimes occurs in early pregnancy, with menstruation. Of course some women do have early morning nausea and indigestion. There are a variety of symptoms of pregnancy which have been popularized in fiction and, in fact, can occur in real life, but often don't. All of this means that the only way to be certain whether you're pregnant or not in the early stages is by medical examination supported by adequate laboratory tests.

Women have always been interested in finding out as soon as possible whether or not they are pregnant, and tests to determine this are not necessarily new. In ancient Egyptian times the women kept a pot of barley seeds and poured some of their urine over the barley each day. If the barley began to sprout the woman was pregnant. This had some scientific basis because the increased amount of hormones in the urine during pregnancy would stimulate the growth of the barley seeds.

SEX VARIETY

Judging by the relatively small number of letters received regarding varieties of sexual expression, one might suspect that they didn't occur very often. However, there is still another interpretation. People who engage in oral sex and other forms of sexual activity really aren't worried very much about it. It is only when they think they are going to have problems that individuals who engage in these forms of sexual activity become concerned.

Dear Dr. Lamb—I am a student at college and to avoid the possibility of pregnancy like many girls at our school I have indulged in oral sex. I am in my third year at school and can truthfully say that no boy has entered my body in regular intercourse. However, information has come to some of us girls that it is possible to get VD in the mouth. Is this possible? I have satisfied my boyfriends by oral means until they have completely ejected themselves. This is a growing activity with young girls and boys. If you could tell us about the possibility of VD, you may be able to help many girls right here in our school.

Comment—It would appear that oral sex is much more common in the younger generation than in older people as a means of sexual expression. A number of popular marriage and sex manuals have advocated it, and many psychiatrists consider it as a normal form of sexual expression.

Yes, it is possible to get venereal disease of the mouth. Syphilis can be transmitted through any moist droplet from an infected person to another person. This can occur (although rarely) even by kissing. Gonorrhea of the throat has been reported in a number of instances, and because of the frequency of oral sex, a number of clinics designed to detect venereal disease now do throat swabs and cultures as well as the traditional examination of the genitalia. The tissues of the throat are somewhat more resistant to gonorrhea than the primary sexual organs, but nevertheless such an infection can occur. Gonorrhea of the rectum is also a possibility in individuals who engage in rectal sex.

Dear Dr. Lamb—Once in the bittersweet past I had an Oriental wife. That lovely wife and I enjoyed our sex and often indulged in oral sex. She was a very clean person and not once was there any offensive odor. Now I am married to a Western wife and she likewise is a very clean person, but I have had her come directly from a bath so hot I could not drink it and found that there was a slight, but very unpleasant odor. If we happen to have sex without a bath first, the odor can be and often is very offensive. I cannot smell it when she is clothed, but with the closeness of the situation it is bad enough that I have never attempted anything like my

39

first wife and I used to enjoy, and I simply cannot. Is there any explanation for this? She is clean.

Comment—Individuals react differently to odors, and part of our reaction to them is no doubt a conditioned or learned response. One of my obstetrician friends has told me that he thinks the upsurge in interest in "feminine hygiene" is directly related to the upsurge in oral sex.

The body normally produces odors which have nothing to do with whether or not a person is clean. There are really two types of sweat glands. One of these produces simple body water or ordinary sweat. The other so-called sweat glands are really "sex glands." In more primitive animals they are used for sexual attraction. These fairly sharp and pungent odors are stronger in some people than in others. The number of these specialized sweat glands has a lot to do with the strength of the odor. The Oriental people have fewer of these specialized sweat glands than do other races. The Caucasian is second with the black race third. Caucasians are sometimes surprised to learn that they have a strong body odor as compared to the Oriental, but it is true. To some people these odors are strongly stimulating sexually. To others they are not. One woman may like the strong musky smell of her man and would rather sleep with him before he showers, and the next woman may be revolted by his odor.

Dear Dr. Lamb—I would like to know if there is any possible damage to a woman if the man has intercourse using her rectum.

Comment—If it is done forcibly or too vigorously, there is always the danger of tearing the muscular sphincter of the anus. This can cause some problems in bowel leakage or bowel incontinence thereafter. Done carefully, this problem need not occur. Another possible problem is a slight cracking or minor tearing of the lining of the anus. The possibility of venereal infection of the rectum is just as real as the possibility of venereal infection from ordinary vaginal sexual relations.

If vaginal penetration follows rectal penetration without proper hygiene, the woman is likely to develop a severe vaginal infection. Although I have never seen it or received any letters on this problem, I was startled recently to learn from a scientific report that it was not too uncommon during rectal activity, particularly between men in a homosexual relationship, for one man to insert his entire fist into the other man's rectum. This, of course, can cause severe damage including laceration of the lower rectum and sigmoid colon as well as tearing the important muscles that control the rectal sphincter.

Dear Dr. Lamb—Would you please advise on the physical problems or repercussions that can come from oral and anal copulation between male and female or male and male sexual relationships and animals and humans also. Can physical harm come from swallowing male sperm?

Comment—It's true that people do everything, and even with animals. The latter, though, is more apt to occur in a rural background where animals are more available. I have already discussed the problems of rectal sex in response to the previous letter and this applies to whether the rectal sex is heterosexual or homosexual. There does not appear to be any physical danger associated with animal-human sexual relationships. In fact it has only been very recently that it has been possible to infect an animal with gonorrhea. The fact that animals appear to be resistant to gonorrhea has made it difficult to do many laboratory studies in animals that would have helped in developing vaccines and other advances that have been achieved with other infectious diseases.

There is no danger in swallowing sperm, as long as the man does not have venereal disease.

Dear Dr. Lamb—I need advice and quickly. My husband and I have been married ten years. For the most part, it has been a very good and normal marriage. We have five wonderful children and what appears to be an ideal home life. I would call it ideal myself except for these few instances which I am writing about. We probably have sex on the average of three or four times a week, sometimes more, sometimes less, depending on circumstances. This is a very good and normal relationship, usually. But once in a while he wants what I consider to be a very deviated relationship. He calls it "playing around." I call it playing around with homosexuality, namely his position is opposite or upside down from mine.

He likes to kiss at the vaginal area and wants me to do the same for him. Once he wanted me to use my hands to bring on his climax and once he even wanted me to use my mouth. I am very disturbed and I get sick at my stomach just thinking about it. This does not happen often. Mostly we have a great relationship with all the normal love play. Does he need counseling or do I? I love him and want to help him if I can.

He has not displayed this urge more than probably a half dozen times in our marriage, but I have a strong feeling it would have happened more often if I would cooperate. He has also admitted to masturbation on a few instances, which I cannot understand since I cannot remember ever refusing him other than these instances which I considered to be abnormal. There is no one else I could ever go to with such a problem, and I am losing respect for him under these conditions.

Comment—There is no way that sex relations of any type between a man and a woman can be classified as a homosexual act. This attitude reflects confusion about the meaning of oral-genital activity. It's quite common for a person to want to enjoy a variety of sexual expressions. This is one way of avoiding "boredom" in marriage. Either early or after the marriage stabilizes, most couples experiment with different forms of sexual expression. A recent survey showed about 50 percent of the doctors polled considered oral-genital sex activity as normal (and incidentally, a high percentage of doctors are relatively conservative about sex).

Kinsey and many biologists who observed that oral-genital activity is common in the animal kingdom and occurs frequently between people consider it entirely normal. The same is true for masturbation. It is true that some individuals don't enjoy these forms of activity and for one reason or another, it is revolting to them. If one of the marriage partners truly doesn't enjoy a particular form of sexual expression, he should tell his partner so and find other ways of mutual satisfaction.

THE LOST CLITORIS

There is still a lot of confusion about the clitoris, even in identifying it.

Dear Dr. Lamb—About five years ago I was dating this guy. I was engaged to him and was very ignorant about sex and still am. I remember that I had this little ball just inside at the top of the labia. I referred to it as my cherry. I knew it has some importance and could not lose it. One night we were sexually playing with each other, but we did not have sex completely. The next night I met him at a reception. I was very sore and hurting so much I didn't know what to do. I could only tell him how I hurt down there. I also noticed that little ball wasn't there any more. I remember looking and feeling for it, but I couldn't find it. I had lost something important. I didn't know how important or what its function was. My inside of the lip sagged more with skin. I looked and felt for about a week, but the little ball never returned. I couldn't go to anyone I was so embarrassed. This may sound silly to you, but I would love to have this experience cleared up. I am married now and have had a hard time for years trying to have a climax and keeping moisture during sex. I want sex but can't get overly

43

stimulated. I would like to know what happened to me during my earlier experience and if this has any bearing on my later sexual life.

Dear Dr. Lamb—Does the fact that my clitoris never erects lessen the pleasure for my companion during the sex act? I have heard there is a condition called a hooded clitoris which can be remedied by minor surgery. Is that true?

Comment—The little ball that the lady thinks she lost is undoubtedly her clitoris. The clitoris is the female equivalent of the penis. It's difficult to identify when it is not stimulated. During sexual excitement it is erected and can readily be identified. It is highly sensitive and if overstimulated, for example by manipulation during sexual activity, it can cause pain and soreness. The fact that she hasn't noticed it since her painful experience suggests that her clitoris has not been erected and that she has not been adequately sexually stimulated since that date. This conclusion is supported by her own description of her inability to be sexually aroused or have an orgasm. All of these factors may be related to her ignorance about sex and the deep impression that her early painful experience may have made, or she may have more deep-rooted problems related to sex. If she understands she didn't lose anything and that the soreness might have been a natural event of early lovemaking perhaps this would help relieve her mind. Nevertheless, she needs to learn to be secure in her sexual relationship and enjoy sexual activity to overcome her "frigidity." This in itself may allow her to enjoy sex and have an erect clitoris. This way she may find her "lost ball."

Whether or not the female clitoris is erected is usually of little consequence to the male in his own personal enjoyment of sex. Many men, however, are unhappy if their companion does not also enjoy sex and feel that it reflects on their ability to induce a proper sexual response in the woman. Women, however, do have orgasms and continue to enjoy sex even if the clitoris has been removed.

44

III

Special Problems of Women

WOMEN HAVE A HOST OF PROBLEMS peculiar to their sexual function. Some of these can be very frightening if they are not understood. Young girls, for example, frequently think that the normal vaginal discharge that first appears at the beginning of their sexually mature years is an indication of venereal disease.

NORMAL DISCHARGE

Dear Dr. Lamb—I am a seventeen-year-old girl and I am very distressed over a vaginal discharge that I have had for some time now. It is quite bothersome and I would like some advice. I have never had sexual intercourse but I do masturbate. The discharge does not look like menstrual blood. It looks like old blood and sometimes has dark brown mucus in it. There is no itching or soreness in my vaginal area. It is not as heavy as my menstrual flow, but sometimes it is heavy enough to come through my panties just enough to make me uncomfortable. What is this condition and what causes it? Is there anything I can do to correct it without going to a doctor? I have no mother and I find it embarrassing to talk about personal things with my father.

45

Dear Dr. Lamb—I am writing you because I have a problem which is very embarrassing for me to talk about to anyone. I am a sixteen-year-old girl and whenever my boyfriend and I "make out" I get a clearish-like discharge in my vagina. This also happens when I'm not with him, such as in school. What could this be? I am worried about it.

Dear Dr. Lamb—I am a teen-age girl. I have not started menstruation yet but I do have a vaginal discharge (I have never noticed any blood in it). I have had it for about a year now and haven't seen a doctor. I would like to know what could be the cause and if it could lead to any serious complication.

Dear Dr. Lamb—There is a seepage of a water-like fluid from my vagina. I noticed that this would happen for a few days after my menstrual period, but now it is continual. I have a doctor's appointment in a few weeks. The doctor said to cancel it if I felt okay and I do feel okay, but if this is serious I guess I'll have to keep it. I am sixteen and very embarrassed about personal problems. I'll die if I have to tell my mom why I am keeping this appointment, and it will be very difficult to tell the doctor.

Dear Dr. Lamb—My thirteen-and-a-half-year-old daughter told me she had a fluid-like substance flowing from her vagina. She hasn't yet started her period. Is this something to worry about? There is no pain or anything wrong in that area.

Comment—The vagina normally secretes a fluid to provide moisture necessary to protect its delicate lining. The normal amount of secretions is sufficiently scant to produce only an occasional stain on the underwear. The amount can be significantly increased by a variety of factors which result in a greater blood flow to the pelvic organs.

The fluid is often whitish in color which gives rise to the

term "leukorrhea" (leuko means white). As the material dries it may cause a brownish-yellow stain. This normal discharge is essentially odorless and doesn't cause itching or irritation. The amount increases markedly at puberty before the time the periods start and for a few years following. The amount gradually decreases and it requires no attention since it's a normal response. An increased discharge often occurs in women who stand for prolonged periods, douche too frequently, or have any other cause for prolonged accumulation of excess amounts of blood in the pelvic area (such as frequent sexual arousal without orgasm). It can also occur as the result of a tear in the cervix which may follow childbirth.

Fluid secretions in the vagina normally increase about midway between the periods. This type of material may not always be whitish, but may more nearly resemble the raw white of an egg and is called mucus. The increased natural lubricant at this point in the menstrual cycle corresponds to the time that the ovum, or egg, is released and ready to be impregnated. The increased lubrication facilitates the sex act.

It is a mistake to use a variety of chemical douches, sprays, and other devices to attempt to eliminate these secretions. A girl at the puberal stage is well advised just to ignore them. If there is any chance that the discharge is related to anything else, of course a medical examination is required to identify the problem. Considering the frequency of gonorrhea these days, a medical examination is a necessity if the girl has been sexually active.

MENSTRUATION

Many young girls are confused about menstruation. This is a very important event in their lives, and you can be sure when this time comes the girls will be exchanging notes. It's difficult to imagine that such an important event would go undiscussed or unquestioned.

Dear Dr. Lamb—I am a young girl, aged eleven. My mom doesn't always tell me things that I want and need to know so I decided to ask you. The first time you menstruate, what does the flow look like? I want to know this because in my underwear there is a dark yellow stain. This started at the beginning of the month. If I'm not menstruating, what is this?

Comment—The normal vaginal discharge is often increased before the onset of periods and for the first few years after the menstrual periods have started. The dried, natural discharge is undoubtedly what this girl is noticing. The menstrual discharge itself, of course, is blood of variable amounts. Characteristically, at the onset of menstruation the amount of bleeding is minimal.

Dear Dr. Lamb—Why is it that about eight to ten days after my period I get this dull ache in my lower side which lasts about twenty-four hours? The ache is a little more severe if I stand.

Comment—This girl is describing the common ovulatory pain. Ovulation occurs at about the midpoint between periods. When it occurs there is often pain in the lower portion of the abdomen, sometimes in the center and other times either to the right or left side. If it happens to be along the right side, it can be confused with appendicitis. It is a normal response and the mid-cycle pain tends to disappear as the girl gets older.

Dear Dr. Lamb—I am writing you about a problem that I've had for thirteen days. My period was late and a friend suggested that I should use turpentine as it always works for her. So I took her advice and took one teaspoon of turpentine mixed with one-half glass of lukewarm water every night before bedtime and every morning before going to school. I tried that for four days and finally my period started. I usually menstruate for four days, but it's been thirteen days and it's still coming. Today it is a bit slower and it goes off and on all day. Please tell me what's the matter. Is there any help for me? I am only fifteen years old and I'm very afraid.

Comment—Irregular menstrual cycles are common, particularly in the first few years that a girl's sexual cycle is being established. Whether the period is early or late is of no particular importance except for those individuals who are using the time of the period in an effort to use the rhythm method of birth control. Preoccupation with regularity in itself causes a girl or woman to be nervous, and the nervousness then can cause irregularity. It becomes somewhat of a vicious cycle. Young girls should be instructed not to try to treat themselves with household remedies for imagined disorders. If there were adequate communication with a knowledgeable parent, most of these problems could be avoided.

Dear Dr. Lamb—I am a fourteen-year-old girl who had sexual intercourse once about four months ago. Since then I have not had a menstrual period. I know I am not pregnant. Do you know what is wrong?

Comment—It's fortunate that she knows she's not pregnant. Not every young girl can be so certain. The early signs of pregnancy may be so minimal that they could be missed. This girl's problem may be the normal irregularity associated with the onset of recurring menstrual cycles. It is not unusual for girls to miss having menstrual periods for several months. It should also be kept in mind that menstrual periods are affected by psychic or emotional factors. If she feels guilty about her sexual experience and is particularly nervous about it, this may well have contributed to anxiety and influenced her menses.

Dear Dr. Lamb—After checking with my doctor I am still concerned over my skipping menstrual periods. I am a healthy woman of twenty-eight who until recently has always been very regular. I did diet over a period of months and lost twenty pounds, but stuck to a good, well-balanced eating routine. Could this have had some effect?

Comment—There are so many causes for menstrual irregularity that it is not possible to pinpoint any one factor and say that's it. The woman who is regular throughout her reproductive years must indeed be a rarity.

It is true that weight reduction, particularly from a severely restricted diet, will affect the sexual functions and could affect one's menstrual cycle. It can also affect a person's sex drive and sexual capacity.

Dear Dr. Lamb—I am a seventeen-year-old girl, and ever since I began menstruating at age fifteen I have never been regular. I skip months now and then. My doctor told me I had anemia and that was why I was always tired. He gave me some iron and thyroid pills, but my father lost his job and I am no longer able to see the doctor. Before I left he gave me some strong liquid iron and told me I would be normal in three weeks and continue my periods. Well, two months later I am still as tired as ever and still without my periods. Could you please give me some advice. I am scared it will affect me and I won't be able to have kids.

Comment—This is the usual irregularity problem again. Anemia is common in women during the childbearing years. The recurrent loss of blood with menstruation can lead to an iron deficiency anemia, unless there is an adequate amount of iron intake in the diet. Women in these years need about twice as much iron as men and post-menopausal women. A simple iron deficiency anemia should have been corrected by the administration of iron. The fact that the girl still complains of fatigue suggests that her difficulties are not solely related to her menstrual periods. There are many causes for fatigue besides female complaints. There are numerous examples of women with generalized fatigue and ill-defined complaints who really have an unsatisfactory sexual life. It is to be expected that a seventeen-year-old girl who is not sexually active is experiencing recurrent sexual frustration. This

50

and other possible causes for fatigue need to be explored.

Dear Dr. Lamb—I am a single girl of twenty-six. Until two years ago my menstrual cycle was normal. Then the periods started getting farther and farther apart. I have skipped three normal periods. Is it possible to have the menopause at twenty-six? I can truthfully say I have not molested my delicate feminine organ with men, pills, or drugs. Should I consult a doctor? I am not worried, but puzzled.

Comment—Rarely women start the change of life in their latter twenties, but this is most unusual. The absence of periods at this age is usually not an indication of the menopause. There are a number of factors which can cause absent periods, and it probably would be a good idea for this individual to visit her doctor.

Dear Dr. Lamb—Is there cause for concern if spotting continues for three days following intercourse which occurred in the middle of the cycle? What are the chances that this may indicate conception has occurred? What other possible causes could there be for this spotting?

Comment—Mid-cycle spotting or bleeding can be a normal event. At the time of ovulation there is a sharp drop in the amount of female hormone produced by the ovary. Immediately thereafter the amount of female hormone produced begins to increase again. Whenever there is an insufficient amount of female hormone, the lining of the womb begins to shed. This sharp decrease in female hormones at the mid-cycle point of ovulation can cause normal mid-cycle bleeding. The fact that this girl had intercourse at the time of the spotting strongly suggests that intercourse occurred near or at the time of ovulation, which of course greatly increases the likelihood that a pregnancy might occur. The spotting itself is not an indication of pregnancy however. Some women interpret this mid-period spotting or flow as a second menstrual period and think they are having two menstrual periods a month.

Dear Dr. Lamb—Is it true a woman has a period of menstruating for thirty years? If she starts at a young age, will she stop earlier or last longer?

Comment—Usually, women who begin menstruating early are the ones who will menstruate the longest. Similarly, women who have a well-adjusted, enjoyable sex life early in life and continue it are the ones who are apt to continue to enjoy an active sexual life into their later years.

Dear Dr. Lamb—Would you please give me some information about menstrual periods during pregnancy? I am two months pregnant and had a regular menstrual period. My doctor says it's normal in some women and not to worry, but I am afraid it might cause trouble with the baby. What do you think?

Comment—I think the lady's doctor is right. It's not rare for a woman to have one or two menstrual cycles after she's pregnant. In much rarer instances, women will continue to have some menstrual flow well into their pregnancy. It is rather difficult to explain why this happens, since there is an increased amount of female hormones present throughout the normal pregnancy.

Dear Dr. Lamb—I am thirty-four years old and would like to know if your menstrual periods change as you get older. I have three children. During the last three months my periods have been terrible. I pass quite a lot of blood clots, and they are big clots, for two days. I usually flood and this goes on for five days altogether. I never had periods like this before and am almost afraid I won't stop flooding. Should I go to a doctor or does this sound normal?

Dear Dr. Lamb—I am twenty years old. My problem is my

52

periods. They have always been normal but I have a lot of cramping. Now my periods are excessive in flow with a lot of clots and usually they last longer than before. Sometimes they last as long as two weeks. This just started about two months ago. Is this normal, or is it a sign that something is wrong?

Comment—Both of these women are complaining about excessive menstrual bleeding. In one instance the flow is very heavy for a normal length of time and in the other instance the bleeding is prolonged. There are many causes for these types of problems and all of them indicate the need for a medical examination, regardless of the age of the woman. In women who are usually somewhat older than either of these two, fibroids or tumors of the uterus can be a cause. Psychological factors, including marital harmony, are also important. Not only may young girls have scanty periods when they first start menstruation, but some of them have excessive flow. This may occur for the first two or three years while the periods are becoming stabilized.

CRAMPS

Dear Dr. Lamb—I have a problem I hope you can help me with. About two years ago I started having very bad menstrual cramps. They are so bad I throw up and spend most of the first day lying in bed crying. Up until that time I wasn't bothered a bit with them and felt women who complained of them were just "faking." Close to the time I started to have the cramps was when I first went "all the way" with my boyfriend. Could this have some relationship to the cramps? What can be done about them? I am twenty-one years old and I hate to think of going through this for the rest of my life. I am really afraid I have hurt myself somehow during sexual intercourse, and that is the reason.

Comment—Painful menstrual cramps are a frequent complaint of young women. It is typical for the major difficulty to occur the first day, as this woman has experienced. Painful menstruation of this type goes under the technical name "dysmenorrhea." It can be very mild or quite severe. Approximately 50 percent of all women experience this type of difficulty between the ages of seventeen and twenty-five. Peculiarly, it doesn't affect girls in the first years of their menstrual cycle, and this particular type of menstrual pain doesn't persist after the mid-twenties.

The cramping pain usually goes away about the time the period starts. It is usually below the navel and may extend down the front of the leg. With the pain the young woman may be pale, nauseated, sick, and sweaty. There is a general opinion that this difficulty seems to be much less common among young women than in the past, and when it does occur it is less severe.

Anxiety does seem to be an important factor, and it could well be that this young lady's anxiety over her previous sexual experience has contributed to the severity of her cramps. This type of menstrual cramping also tends to disappear after a pregnancy. When the pains are severe, the best thing to do is to take some medicine which affords some pain relief (usually aspirin is a good choice). Rest and relaxation and sometimes the use of a hot-water bottle over the lower part of the abdomen are helpful. Doctors do not like to give strong drugs for a disorder of this type which occurs each month. The person can become dependent on the drugs and this can cause additional problems. Exercise is recommended as one way of minimizing the problem and it seems to help some girls. When the case is unusually severe, I recommend that the girl be seen by a gynecologist to be certain that there are no other contributing factors. Understanding and sympathetic support are also helpful. Removing undue concern about sexual problems and anxieties is often indicated. Regardless of the severity of the menstrual cramps, they have nothing to do with causing any problems with subsequent pregnancies.

Masters and Johnson have shown that the pain can be relieved by an orgasm. After an orgasm the excess blood causing congestion of the sex organs drains out of the pelvis. This observation suggests the pain is related to congestion caused by unrelieved sexual tension.

Dear Dr. Lamb—I am twenty-eight and am overweight. I've been that way all my life, and I'm a borderline diabetic. Otherwise I'm in good health. My problem is that I have considerable trouble with my periods. About a year and a half ago I went to a female specialist for a physical. Everything was okay. He seemed to think my cramping was caused by nerves. I took a tranquilizer for about six months but this didn't seem to help.

Lately the pain has become so severe that I've been taking Darvon compound. I can't even wear a tampon anymore. I always wore them until a few months ago. Then knife-sharp pains started when I was using them. Now I have the pains no matter what I do. Sometimes they are so severe I have to hold on to a chair or the wall to keep from falling. I feel weak for a couple of days after my period. I have had two children, ages ten and four. I've never used birth control medicines, so you can plainly see that I don't conceive easily. The doctor couldn't find any reason for my problem and said everything was okay.

I can't stand or sit during my periods without these stabbing pains. This never happened before until my last child was born. I never had any discomfort before then. Is this normal for my age group and what can I do? I am dreading my next period. Each one gets worse.

Comment—Severe menstrual cramps seen in women past twenty-five years of age are different from those seen in younger women. They may occur just preceding the period and be relieved by the menstrual flow, or as in this woman's case, they can occur throughout the period and even last for a short time afterwards. Fortunately, this form of menstrual pain is less common than that noted in younger women.

55

There are many things which can cause it, including anxiety. Clearly this woman's doctor thought that might be a factor in her case, as indicated by her letter. Anything which contributes to congestion or increased amount of blood in the pelvic region seems to contribute to this problem. A pelvic infection, family problems, or too sedentary a life may all be contributing factors. Occasionally the accumulation of fluid associated with "pre-menstrual tension" is the cause, and helping to relieve this problem will also alleviate part of the painful cramping difficulty.

PREMENSTRUAL TENSION

Dear Dr. Lamb—I am forty-three years old and don't think I am old enough to go through the change of life, but when it comes time for my period, I get so sick and depressed I just want to hide from everyone. My feet swell, I have headaches, which is something I never had before, the worst part is I nearly go blind and my eyes bother me so. I have glasses but they don't help. Mornings when I get up my eyes are nearly swollen shut. What could cause this?

Dear Dr. Lamb—I retain so much extra water in my tissues that I gain about four to five pounds of water and my breasts hurt so bad I can't sleep on my stomach or let my husband even touch them. If I bump them accidentally, it really hurts. They swell up about one to one and a half inches. The rest of my body swells also but it doesn't hurt. The swelling lasts about two and a half weeks, and as soon as my periods start, it ends. Then it begins a few days after my period is over, so I only have about ten days without it.

This problem started when I was on the pill, so my doctor switched pills and that didn't help. Then I stopped the pill and I still have the problem. I've taken water pills and as long as I'm taking them it seems to help, but there's no way of telling whether I'm eliminating too much. I've had a thyroid test and it shows that I don't have any problem.

Comment—Both of these women are explaining the typical problems of accumulation of fluid and premenstrual tension. Women commonly have a change in personality and disposition just preceding the menses. They are often more irritable, have headaches, and complain of fatigue at this time. As women get older these problems tend to become more severe. The female hormones increase progressively from the end of one menstrual period to the next and are related to the retention of fluid. In many women the fluid retention phase is limited to a few days immediately preceding the menses, but longer periods of fluid retention are not uncommon, particularly as women get older.

The use of medicines to cause the kidneys to flush out salt (the sodium in the salt) which carries the excess water with it often relieves the symptoms. The problem is that these pills, in washing out salt, also will wash out other minerals, particularly potassium. The rapid loss of sodium and potassium salts may cause fatigue. Women with this problem are well advised to limit their intake of salt, particularly for the ten-day period preceding their menses.

FAINTING

Dear Dr. Lamb—I have a sixteen-year-old girl who is active in sports and is in the marching band at her school. She is in good health most of the time. However, sometimes when she is menstruating she has what she calls the tingles. She feels numb all over and has trouble breathing and sometimes faints. These attacks usually occur after some exertion, either marching or playing softball or other sports.

Two doctors have seen her during these attacks, and they both say this is normal in teen-age girls during this time of the month. However, no other girls we know have this problem. The doctors say this is hyperventilation.

Does this happen to a lot of girls? Also, do they get over it when they become adults? Is there any medicine that can be taken to prevent this?

Comment—Sweating, nausea, and a faint feeling commonly occur in young women during the first day of their menstrual period. It is most prevalent in women between the ages of seventeen and twenty-five. Apparently this girl is having additional problems other than those that occur simply with menstruation. Hyperventilation refers to overbreathing and it most often occurs when a person is nervous or experiencing anxiety. The overbreathing causes the lungs to blow off too much carbon dioxide and upsets the chemical balance of the body. This then causes the tingling feeling in the fingers, arms, and sometimes around the lips. It goes away if the individual will control the breathing and breathe shallowly at a slow rate. Overbreathing, or hyperventilation, can contribute to a sense of faintness or can actually induce fainting. It is likely that this girl is experiencing anxiety with her period, and since she is more susceptible to fainting at that time anyway, the hyperventilation has a more marked effect.

SEX DURING PERIODS

Dear Dr. Lamb—I would like to know if it is safe for two people to have sexual relations during the woman's menstrual period. Are there any detrimental effects involved where the couple has sexual intercourse during the menstrual period if she uses a rubber diaphragm to prevent the flow temporarily?

Comment—If by safe a person means free of harmful physical effects, there is no reason to be concerned about having sexual intercourse during the menstrual period. The menstrual flow is not infectious, and there is no reason to believe that the sexual activity will cause infection in the woman either. There is really no point in using a rubber diaphragm during the menstrual period. Masters and Johnson have shown quite clearly that with the change in the size of the vaginal canal during the sex act, even a well-fitted diaphragm no longer fits. In other words the diaphragm does very little to produce a mechanical blockage.

HYGIENE DURING PERIODS

Dear Dr. Lamb—Could you tell me if it is harmful to wash one's hair during one's period. I wash mine every other night because it gets extremely oily and my scalp itches me to death. During my period Mom will not let me wash it, and the kids at school tease me about it. Some other girls have the same problem, but their hair does not get as dirty in one week as mine will in two days. If it is not harmful, please let me know so I can show this to my mother.

Comment—There seems to be an old wives' tale that washing the hair during the menstrual period will cause some disastrous consequence. There is not one bit of truth in this notion, and it's perfectly all right for a girl to wash her hair, bathe or exercise during her menstrual period.

DOUCHING

A woman's natural desire for cleanliness and her concern about the possibilities of an infection often lead her to feel that douching is necessary. Most doctors feel that it is not necessary unless a woman has a medical problem or an infection that requires it.

Dear Dr. Lamb—You've probably never been asked this question before. It's very important to me. My boyfriend and I have been having sexual relations since last summer. What I want to know is exactly what is douching and how to do it. I am so afraid of contracting a disease or an infection if I don't, but it is next to impossible to hide those things available at drugstores. Hiding a small bottle of pills is one thing, but all of the douches seem to be large cans. Is there anything at home that can be used?

Is it necessary? I'd hate to create and give him something. What happens if I don't douche? Is it necessary to use a product from the drugstore, and if so, which type should a teen-age girl use and how often? I'll only have intercourse once or twice a month.

Comment—This girl touches on most of the concerns about douching. In the first place, nature has provided its own cleansing mechanism, and that's the natural flow of lubricants in the vagina. An adequate amount of cleanliness is provided by ordinary bathing of the genitalia. This isn't going to satisfy some women, however, and they still want to douche regardless of what they're told. For those who must douche, it's important that they use a very mild douche. The vagina normally is acid, which helps protect it against a number of different types of bacteria. Washing out the vaginal cavity may actually make it more susceptible to an infection.

The best douche fluid to use is one that approximates the normal chemistry of body fluids. This is a mild salt water. To a quart of water that is comfortably warm, a person can add two or three teaspoons of salt and no more. In rinsing out the vaginal vault, no excessive pressure should be used. To avoid this, the douche should be accomplished with a douche bag and not a bulb. The bag shouldn't be hung up high to induce pressure, but should be held at arm's length or hung no higher than shoulder level. Of course, the nozzle should be clean before using and you should never use a nozzle that someone else has used because that's a good way to spread disease.

Douching is not a preventive of venereal disease. People get venereal disease by having sexual relations with someone who has it. Although personal hygiene is desirable, it is not true that lack of it alone causes venereal disease. One can get some protection from venereal disease, certainly, by immediately cleansing oneself after sexual relations, but this is a highly unreliable method of prevention.

Douching is of little value in preventing pregnancies. After all, the initial drops of semen contain the largest amounts of sperm cells. These can move rather quickly into the uterus, long before a woman will have time to jump out of bed and douche. Besides, the sexual act is not necessarily complete nor are the partners fulfilled immediately at the time of orgasm. It is not very conducive to a satisfying sexual life to be jumping in and out of bed and grabbing the douche bag instantaneously at the end of the sex act.

One should never use any strong chemical for a douche. The only time a woman should use a douche besides the mild salt water mentioned above should be under a doctor's direction. He may prescribe a vinegar douche for an infection of the vagina. Some of the other chemicals may irritate the vagina and make it susceptible to infection. If an infection is already present, the doctor needs to identify what is causing it, and administering a strong chemical douche makes diagnosis more difficult.

Dear Dr. Lamb—My doctor tells me to douche as little as possible. Other doctors recommend douching frequently. The writing on my douche powder container states never to douche more than twice a week, yet my marriage manual states to douche often and after each intercourse. Why is there such a difference of opinion by doctors? What are the effects of douching that call for such diverse opinions? Can douching be harmful?

Comment—The reason there is such a widespread difference of opinion is because of the widespread degree of ignorance. The difference in opinion, however, may not be as great as it seems. Douches are sometimes properly recommended when a woman has a vaginal infection. Otherwise, they don't have much to offer. Marriage manuals are notoriously inaccurate.

Dear Dr. Lamb—Will you please write something about women douching. I have a twenty-one-year-old daughter, but still do not know when a girl should start douching. My daughter thought she had to start when she was nineteen and made her first visit for a smear test which she has twice a year. During my married life my husband seemed to think it dried a woman out, and I would have trouble. A doctor told me to have him use a lubricant. He did once, but no more.

My husband feels so strongly about women not douching that he would probably blame me if he knew his daughter was doing it, and thinking of her future marriage would probably want me to discourage her. A man can never know how a woman has to feel clean because he doesn't have the secretions she has, especially before and after her period. And let's face it, married life gives her more secretions. I don't feel clean, no matter how much I bathe. What are the best ingredients for a douche powder?

Comment—This lady's husband obviously has a lot of good common sense. The secretions that a woman has are her normal lubricants. Washing out the vaginal vault can lead to it being drier and can minimize the available lubricant for sexual activity. It is true that married life gives a woman more secretions, but that's nature's way of helping the woman to be better able to engage effectively in an active sex life. As I mentioned in answer to the previous letters, the best douche for normal women, if they insist on using one, is a mild warm saltwater solution.

TAMPONS

Dear Dr. Lamb—I am writing to ask you about a topic I know very little about, and I'm sure other girls are in the same predicament. My mother was shocked when I asked her and wouldn't discuss it, and my best friend is as uninformed as I am.

Would you say something about tampons? My mother indicated that only married women can wear them (implying that virgins cannot), but I know several girls who do and I feel sure that they are virgins as I am. Who exactly can wear them? Can they go up into you any further than you put them? How are they worn and how long? How can a person choose one among the many brands on the market? What is the difference between super and regular sizes?

Also, does wearing tampons make it seem like you're not a virgin? My friend's mother said this and won't let her wear them.

Comment—A woman needs to wear some sort of protection in order to absorb the menstrual flow. This can be either an external pad or an internal pad. The tampon is literally an internal pad, inserted into the vagina to absorb the menstrual flow.

Lots of people think that virgins cannot wear tampons. The assumption is that the hymen membrane has sealed off the opening, and to wear a tampon it would have to be perforated. The truth is that many virgins have enough perforation of the hymen that they can use a tampon without difficulty. If the hymen is not at least partially perforated, it will block the menstrual flow and require a minor surgical correction to permit normal menses. If a small-sized virgin is going to use a tampon, she'll want to use the smallest size available and incidentally, the difference between super and regular is merely a matter of size.

It is fair to say that if a girl uses a large tampon over a period of time this will contribute to relaxing her vaginal canal and increasing the size of the normal hymen perforation, even if she is a virgin. This can be beneficial, since for a woman to enjoy sexual relations without pain her vaginal canal must be dilated and her hymen stretched. It's absolutely ridiculous to think that a girl should approach sexual intercourse suddenly without having taken measures to keep her from being hurt and perhaps being permanently psychically traumatized about sexual relations. If the wearing of tampons helps to prepare a woman for an active sex life, it merely helps accomplish what the doctor often advises or initiates in the form of exercises at premarital counseling. This is a lot more important than some figmentary concept about virginity.

Some doctors feel that painful intercourse is less common

now in young women and credit the use of tampons for the improvement.

Dear Dr. Lamb—During the summer months many women are on their periods. Will you tell me if it is safe to wear a napkin while swimming? If not, what should you do when you've just learned to swim and love it and you can't wear tampons?

Comment—It's perfectly safe as far as health is concerned, although it might not be the most aesthetic thing to do. Most women who, for one reason or another, do not use tampons refrain from swimming, at least in a public pool, during their menstrual period.

HONEYMOON CYSTITIS

Dear Dr. Lamb—My husband and I have been married four months, and I have been taking oral contraceptives for about four and a half months. I would guess that I have had this problem I'm writing about for about two and a half months. I did not have it when we got married. Sometimes the following morning after having had sexual intercourse with my husband, I find that I have a continuous "feeling" to urinate, yet I don't need to. When I do try to urinate I get a sensation of discomfort and almost pain. I notice this particularly after a night of prolonged and very active sex. I know it can't be irritation because I am not dry.

I had a premarital checkup four and a half months ago and I had my blood checked about one and a half months ago for venereal disease. About a year ago I was checked by a kidney doctor for one thing or another. In all cases I proved to be all right, but this bothers me for I don't think I should be affected like this. My husband is several years older than I, and I am not quite twenty-one. Is something wrong?

Comment—This is a classic example of "honeymoon cystitis." It can occur in relationship to regular sexual activity

64

whether or not the honeymoon is still on. Women are particularly susceptible to urinary tract infections during their most sexually active years. The outlet tube from the bladder, or urethra, is quite short in the female. It is very easy for bacteria to enter the short urethral tube and also invade the bladder. I am not referring to a venereal infection, but rather any of the host of bacteria that are normally present over the skin and around the female genitals. The mechanical act of sexual intercourse can implant the bacteria right at the opening of the urethral tube.

Another cause of cystitis is the mechanical irritation of the urethral tube. The opening of the urethra, after all, is just above the vaginal opening. During sex the urethral opening may actually be pressed against the pubic bone, caught between the penis and the pubis. Repeated vigorous sexual activity can mechanically irritate the urethral opening. This makes it easier for it to become infected, or it can cause burning on urination and other symptoms associated either with mechanical irritation or bacterial inflammation.

At the time of the honeymoon the increase in vigorous sexual activity often causes both mechanical irritation of the urethral opening and introduces some bacteria into the opening which can cause a urinary tract infection, or cystitis; hence, the term, "honeymoon cystitis." Medical examination and appropriate medication are indicated. A second factor which is helpful, particularly if the irritation is just mechanical, is altering slightly the position for intercourse. By changing the angle of insertion so there will be limited or no pressure upon the urethra, much mechanical irritation can be avoided.

IV

Birth Control and Abortions

IF ALL PREGNANCIES were the result of a desire for a child rather than a desire for sex, there would be a lot fewer people on this earth. A study by Dr. Ann Cartwright reported that about half of Britain's mothers had an unplanned-for and unwanted child. Her study showed that only 54 percent of the mothers surveyed were not using any form of birth control at the time they got pregnant and were happy with having a child. This also indicates that a large percentage of the women were using some form of birth control which proved to be ineffective. In many countries of the world voluntary abortion is the main method of birth control. Certainly family planning is an important issue in the new marriage, or for that matter, between couples who are not married. It is not surprising that many letters are received from people concerned about the problem of birth control and abortion.

There is widespread misinformation and lack of information on these problems despite their importance to individuals' private lives. It is also interesting to note that intelligent, sexually active women do not always use the best forms of birth control. Dr. Takey Christ of the University of North Carolina reported that in a survey of 393 sexually active women nearly sixty-five percent of them used "high-risk" birth control methods. Actually 17 of the group used nothing at all. Another 134 women relied on the withdrawal tech-

66

nique, while 76 used the rhythm method and 7 depended on douching. None of these methods is considered to be very reliable in preventing pregnancy.

FEMALE STERILIZATION

Dear Dr. Lamb—I am expecting my second child in December, to be delivered by cesarean section. My doctor suggests that since this is my second cesarean, I should have my tubes tied. I would like to have this done, but I would like some details about it. How will this affect my period? Is there a chance I could ever get pregnant?

Comment—A tubal ligation is one of the most successful forms of birth control. Its one big disadvantage is that it should be considered as permanent and used only for women who definitely are not planning to have any more children. A good number of women change their minds about this and decide later, for a variety of reasons, that they would like to have another child.

To understand the procedure it is necessary to appreciate the characteristics of the female reproductive system. The uterus is like a large avocado. The stem end of the avocado is similar to the cervix, and the large rounded body of the avocado is comparable to the body of the uterus. Near the top of the body of the uterus on each side is a long narrow tube. These end in a large, mouthlike opening. The ovaries are not very far away from the mouthlike openings. When the egg is released from an ovary, it passes across this space and enters the mouth of one tube. The egg then journeys down the tube and if it meets a sperm, whammo! A pregnancy occurs. The fertilized egg then migrates on down the tube into the body of the uterus where it implants and pregnancy begins.

The tubal ligation merely blocks the tubes so that no egg can get down the tube to meet the sperm. In the classic tubal ligation, an incision is made along the side of the abdomen, the tube is exposed, a section of it is cut out, and the severed ends of the tube are tied off. This in no way interferes with the function of the ovaries, or, for that matter, the function of the uterus. It just mechanically interrupts the passageway that the egg would normally take to reach the uterus. The ovary will continue to produce eggs and will have its normal ovarian function. The uterus will continue to respond normally to the hormone functions of the ovary. For this reason a woman continues to ovulate and she continues to menstruate. She will also have a normal menstrual cycle just the same as she would have if her tubes had been left intact.

Now, what are the chances of getting pregnant after such a procedure? There is some difference in the statistics presented by different people, but for the standard procedure that I have described above, Dr. Charles H. DeBrovner, obstetrician at the New York University School of Medicine in New York City, states that the failure rate is about one in 300 operations for women who have this procedure done at some time after they have recovered from a pregnancy. The failure rate is as high as one in 50 for women who have this procedure done as part of a cesarean section. The U.S. Food and Drug Administration's 1969 report stated that less than one in 200 women got pregnant in any one year after tubal ligation. Nothing in this world is certain, including tubal ligations.

Dear Dr. Lamb—Is it possible for a woman to become pregnant after having her tubes tied? I have heard of a few cases in which this has happened. Please explain. Also, what happens to the eggs when the tubes are tied? Does this cause a delay in the menopause?

Comment—Nothing happens to the woman at all. The eggs are merely absorbed by the body and this creates no problem. Tying of the tubes in no way influences the menopause. In the rare cases of failure in the tubal ligation procedure, apparently the tubes managed to reconnect automatically. After all, nature designed the body to correct any injuries such as a tear, cut, or broken bone. It's not too surprising that the body has resources to correct an injury to the reproductive system, which is what a tubal ligation really is.

Dear Dr. Lamb—If a pregnancy does occur after a tubal ligation, could this cause defective children?
Comment—No, as long as the egg is normal and the sperm is normal, and they meet to produce a pregnancy which is properly nourished in the uterus, the child will be normal.

Dear Dr. Lamb—I had a child by cesarean section nine years ago and at the time I had my tubes tied. Is it possible I can get pregnant? One of my friends had the same operation done and she is seven months pregnant.
Comment—This verifies the remarks I just made. There are occasional instances in which even tubal ligation does not prevent pregnancy, but these are rare cases. The failure rate is greater for tubal ligations that are done in conjunction with a cesarean section. Some obstetricians feel the failure rate is as high as one in fifty in this setting.

Dear Dr. Lamb—I am a young career woman thirty years old. I am considering marriage to a man of thirty-seven. What I want to know is if it's possible for a single woman to have a sterilization operation performed? You see, I don't wish to have children. I have felt this way since I was a teen-ager, and if I'm not able to know my own mind on this subject by now I doubt that I ever would. I can't really take the pill because of the discomfort it causes me, and it increases the clotting of my blood. I wish to be sterilized so there could be no possibility of an accidental pregnancy and so I wouldn't have to risk taking the pill.
Comment—It's a good idea to postpone having any sterilization operation until a person is actually married. If for any reason the marriage doesn't occur, it's entirely possible that if the woman later decides to marry another man, he might wish to have children.

69

Sterilization is legal in all fifty states. Utah was the last state to require that a medical reason must exist for the procedure. In almost all states the decision is between the woman and her doctor.

Dear Dr. Lamb—I am a mother of six children and am taking the pill, and I'm tired of it. A friend of mine just told me of a new operation which they do in a day. They make a small cut near the navel and use a new kind of instrument to go in and cut your tubes. Is this operation in the experimental stage or is it being done in different parts of the country? Also, how much does this operation cost and what are the risks? Where can this be done and also what kind of a doctor would I contact? My doctor is of my faith and will not discuss any form of birth control other than the pills and rhythm method. My husband is a barber and we can't afford any lengthy stay in the hospital.

Comment—New operations are being developed regularly for female sterilization. One operation is much as described. A small incision is made to introduce a very small instrument, or tube, used to pump air into the abdomen. This separates the abdominal organs so they can be seen easily. Then through a second small puncture wound a lighted instrument is passed into the abdomen and through a telescopic device the tubes are located. With electrical current, a section of the tube is coagulated or sealed. This coagulated or sealed section is then cut through to produce the tubal ligation. After the operation is over, the skin incision is so small that it usually doesn't even need a stitch and can be covered with a band-aid. For this reason, it is sometimes called "band-aid" or "belly button" surgery.

The actual operation only lasts approximately twenty minutes. At the North Carolina Memorial Hospital in Chapel Hill it is common for the patient to be admitted overnight, have the surgery the next morning, and be home at noon for lunch or engage in any other activity that she may desire.

70

The procedure is called a laparoscopy tubal sterilization. A similar procedure can be done using a vaginal instead of abdominal approach. One of these projects is underway with Dr. William Little of the University of Miami School of Medicine. At the Surgicenter in Phoenix, Arizona, the laparoscopic sterilization requires a maximum stay of three hours. They are also performed by the St. Luke's Hospital in Kansas City on an out-patient basis.

It's difficult to be specific about the cost, but it's usually cheaper than the classic form of tubal ligation. In many instances it will be below the Blue Cross and Blue Shield payment for hospital costs and surgical fees for sterilization procedures.

As far as the effectiveness of this procedure is concerned, it has not been in use long enough to provide a definitive answer as to whether it will be as effective as the standard, long-used Pomeroy method of tubal ligation I have already described. The only way that the effectiveness of any procedure can be evaluated is over a period of time, but there is no reason to think that the newer procedures of tubal ligation won't be approximately as effective as the earlier methods. Time alone will substantiate or refute this opinion.

Dear Dr. Lamb—Six years ago when my last baby was born by cesarean operation, I had my tubes tied and since then I haven't had any interest in sexual intercourse. Could you please say what might have gone wrong in the operation. I should mention that this was my seventh child and the last two were cesarean, and that's the reason I had my tubes tied.

Comment—There are many reasons for women to lose their interest in sexual activity, and men too for that matter. The fact that it occurred after tubal ligation in no way proves that the tubal ligation had anything to do with the change in the level of sex desire. If a woman loses her interest in sexual life after tubal ligation, it is probably caused by some other factor which may be related to the characteristics of her sex

71

life or her home situation or any of the countless factors which affect a woman's desire or lack of desire.

Dear Dr. Lamb—I am a woman of thirty-five and have remarried. About fourteen years ago I had my tubes tied, but now my husband would like to have a child of his own. I have seven of mine, but I would like to have one for him. We have been married for six years. I was told that I could never have another child, but isn't there something that could be done to change this so that I may have a child at this time?

Dear Dr. Lamb—After my second child was born five years ago, I had my tubes cut, but now that I have lost both of my children, I would like to know if there is any possible way to have another child. I am twenty-five years old, if this will help. This is very important to me.

Comment—In a new marriage a woman may wish to have children. Or, the loss of a child may cause a couple to want more children. Operations are done to try to reconnect the tubes. The reported success is variable. The technique has even been done using a microscope to identify the fine structures and put them together. With the latter technique a success of 25 percent is claimed, with several pregnancies having occurred. Even if the tubes are successfully reconnected, this doesn't always guarantee that a woman is going to be able to have children again, simply because she is getting older by the time she comes to the decision she would like to have more children. While many older women do get pregnant, it's easier when you're younger. I have received a number of letters from women who have had this operation who state that they are now sorry about the whole thing.

MALE STERILIZATION (Vasectomy)

Dear Dr. Lamb—My husband has been considering having

a vasectomy done, but can't understand how he can have the same sensation in having an orgasm when the seminal fluid is not propelled out of the body. Could you explain this?

Comment—There are many misconceptions about the vasectomy operation. To understand the operation one needs to have a little knowledge of the male reproductive tract. The sperm cells are formed in the body of the testicles. Then they migrate to the center of the body of the testicle and eventually all of them are collected into one giant tube which leaves the testicle and passes with the cord from the testicle up to the region of the prostate. This tube is called the vas deferens. It passes through the prostate gland and empties into the urethra, a tube that extends out the shaft of the penis. The urethra is the tube connected to the bottom of the bladder to drain the urine. The prostate is wrapped around the urethra at its beginning, just under the bladder. Multiple openings in the sponge-like prostrate gland drain its secretions into the urethra, near the spot where the vas deferens empties sperm cells into it.

The vasectomy involves a short incision in the scrotum through which the vas deferens tube is found and a segment of this tube is cut out and the free ends are tied off. This essentially interrupts or blocks the tube for the passage of the sperm. This does not mean that the testicles quit producing sperm.

The testicles have two functions: one is to produce sperm, and the other is to produce male hormone. The two are not the same. The cells that produce the male hormone, testosterone, continue to be just as active after the tube has been cut and tied off as they were before.

The semen which is produced during an orgasm contains a lot more than the sperm cells. These, in fact, are just a very small contribution to the volume of the semen. The major portion of semen comes from the prostatic fluids formed by the prostate gland and a considerable quantity from the seminal vesicles. These are two saddlebag-like pouches that extend off the prostate gland and form secretions for the ejaculation. The seminal vesicles, incidentally, are not there for the storage of sperm. They merely produce more fluid for the orgasm. Therefore, after a vasectomy a man continues to have an orgasm which is essentially no different than that which he had experienced before the operation as far as he is concerned. If the operation has been successful, there are no sperm cells present on microscopic examination.

Dear Dr. Lamb—I am a very badly hurt mother. I would like to know whether having an operation to prevent having children will harm a man's married life so that he and his wife can't have any sexual relations. I have heard that it does and that they cannot have intercourse at all. I would like to know if this is true and what effect it has on their health. I have a boy twenty-three years old who had this done. He is a good boy, he never drank, he hates liquor, and he never smoked in his life, and I have to this day never heard him use a dirty or curse word. I am so worried and hurt.

Comment—Normal sexually adequate men without any psychological difficulty are not thought to have any difficulties with sexual relations after a vasectomy. Reactions such as exemplified by this letter are typical of the confusion concerning vasectomies. It is not the same thing as castration or removing of the testicles, and incidentally, even men who have had their testicles removed after achieving sexual maturity often are still able to have sexual intercourse, even though their sex drive may be considerably less than it was before.

Dear Dr. Lamb—In discussing vasectomies with friends who have had them, we have discovered that some men have only soreness in their recovery period while others experience considerable pain, stomach cramps, and backache. Is there a medical reason to explain the difference between these two extremes? Or does the difference lie in the skill of the physician or the type of procedure?

74

Comment—There is a great deal of human variation involved in the recovery from almost any medical procedure. The possibility of postoperative infection is another variable. The scrotum is none too clean and it's difficult to get it adequately sterile for operative procedures.

Most men do better if they will take the time for the first day at least to rest and get off their feet. This helps to decrease the engorgement with blood in the scrotal area. Blood, like any other liquid, runs downhill. The blood from the heart runs downhill to the legs and scrotum, and the way to decrease the pressure at the bottom of the hill is to decrease the height of the hill. Or in other words, when you're lying down there's not much pressure for the blood to run down into the scrotum and cause distention. Staying off the feet and lying down for the remainder of the first day and night after the procedure is a useful approach.

Dear Dr. Lamb—My boyfriend and I are having a conflict. He wants to get fixed so that after we get married he won't have kids for a few years. I want kids. I am trying to explain to him that once he gets fixed, he can't get unfixed. Am I right?

Comment—That's the right attitude because a lot of vasectomies cannot be reversed. There are variable claims on the success of reversal, and no doubt it's partly dependent upon how much of the vas tube was taken out at the time of surgery. A good general figure, though, is only about 25 percent of them can be undone, so the boyfriend in this case would only have about a 25 percent chance of getting "unfixed." Some surgeons claim better success, but the demonstration of sperm cells alone after a corrective operation doesn't necessarily prove that the man will have enough sperm to induce pregnancy. And after all, that's what the whole game's about.

Dear Dr. Lamb—I am on the pill and have two children, but do not desire to become pregnant again. I have read a bit about vasectomies for men. I questioned my

75

husband on having this operation and his attitude was negative. He will not give me any substantial answer to back up his negative attitude. I think he feels if he has this done he will become impotent or less masculine. I've tried to explain that I don't see how this could be. Could you give me some information on how many men have had this done and if they feel impotent or less masculine afterwards. Also, I would like to know how effective it is compared to the pill. I'd want to be reassured of not getting pregnant. Even if he had the operation, I'd probably keep on taking my pills because I'd want to be assured of having my period every twenty-eight days, and if I stopped I wouldn't be sure of that.

Comment—It is probably not a good idea for a wife to push her husband into having a vasectomy. It should be a mutual decision. There is no reason a vasectomy should cause a man to become impotent. There are cases on record of this happening, but usually it is because of psychological factors. If the man does not understand the operation and thinks it's going to affect his masculinity, his lack of confidence may cause exactly that to happen. This is one reason why it's extremely important that a man understand exactly what a vasectomy is and even more important, what it is not.

The Midwest Population Center in Chicago received answers to questionnaires from 320 people who had received vasectomies. It's interesting that 70 percent of the couples claimed that their sex life was better after the operation. Another 20 percent said that it was unchanged, and over 90 percent of the men stated that they felt just as masculine as ever. Another 6 percent of the men stated that they felt more masculine than before the operation.

Some family service groups, however, have reported difficulties. In general, family problems that existed before the operation persisted and sometimes worsened, which simply means that the vasectomy is not an operation to correct family problems. It is likely that most of the adverse effects that occur in men after a vasectomy are related to incomplete understanding of the nature of the operation and psychological problems. It's a good idea to have a psychiatric interview before the surgery if feasible.

Dear Dr. Lamb—I would like to know if a vasectomy would help a man seventy-eight years of age as far as sex is concerned.

Comment—It's a good bet that this man is having trouble with impotence or in maintaining an erection. The vasectomy was once used for this purpose but its effectiveness for this problem is doubtful. It should be used only for the purposes of preventing pregnancies. It should not be expected to accomplish more.

Dear Dr. Lamb—I had a vasectomy six years ago and it was a complete procedure. I saw the two pieces of removed tubing. Recently I had a sperm count and was amazed that it showed positive for sperm. I thought someone had goofed in the laboratory. A second specimen and then a third confirmed the original count. Nowhere had I ever heard that vasectomies can naturally heal, thus allowing sperm to pass completely through the tube as before. Any comments you have on this would be appreciated by all of us who used to think vasectomies were 100 percent.

Comment—It's a good general rule in life not to count on anything being 100 percent, and vasectomies are no exception. One factor which is related to the effectiveness is how the procedure is done. One report by Dr. Hjalmar Carlson, a urologist in Kansas City, states that using an early procedure common at the end of World War II, he observed a reopening of the tube in about 6 percent of the cases. By contrast, in a procedure which removed considerably more tube in a subsequent 1000 cases, he did not experience this problem. The way the vas doubles back on itself next to the testicle, it is possible for the head of the tube near the body of the testicle to unite with a part of the tube past where the cut has been made. In other words, it forms a detour and provides a new channel for the sperm to pass. This complication is relatively rare, but it can and does happen.

Dear Dr. Lamb—I would like to know if there is any connection between a man having a vasectomy and not going bald. I have heard that this is true. A health magazine stated that castrated males produce less androgens (male hormones) and did not become bald, and I wondered if a vasectomy would have the same effect on baldness.

Comment—It is usually said that castrates do not become bald, but that's not universally true. Even women can and do become bald. Vasectomies are not castration, and have no effect on baldness.

THE RHYTHM METHOD

Dear Dr. Lamb—This is a very serious problem, and I'm sure disillusions many other people as well as myself, so I want you to give me a clear-cut, honest answer. My problem concerns the rhythm method of contraception. I was led to believe that the period of time between menstruation and ovulation (roughly fourteen days depending on the length of the entire cycle) was the time when the girl was relatively safe from pregnancy—that is, the egg was still in the ovary and therefore unfertilizable. What's more, the sperm can only survive for about twenty-four hours once inside the womb. I work with a friend, however, who has had the third child "accidentally" and claims there is no such thing as the rhythm method. Could you set me straight?

Dear Dr. Lamb—Could you please tell me if there is really a safe period or how to figure one out? I tried the rhythm method and it didn't work, so now I hope you can give me some advice. I'm forty-seven and my husband is fifty-three, and at this age we wouldn't like to

78

have any more children. I already have seven. I was told that at my age I didn't have to worry, but I'm afraid to take that chance.

Dear Dr. Lamb—I understand that a woman is sterile twelve days before her period, and intercourse can take place without the danger of pregnancy. I usually have a period every twenty-six days, but I see that I am a week over. My husband and I had sex on one of these twelve so-called safe days. Now I'm beginning to wonder if this was really wise. We weren't planning on another child.

Comment—Unfortunately, the rhythm method is based on an idealized concept, as opposed to reality. This doesn't mean it's totally ineffective, but it does mean it has definite limitations. In a study by Drs. Brayer, Chiazze, and Duffy of 2,316 women having 30,655 cycles, it was demonstrated that only 30 percent of the women were truly regular enough to make the rhythm method work. Ideally, a woman ovulates at the midpoint between her periods, and if she has a twenty-eight-day menstrual cycle, this means ovulation occurs on the fourteenth day. Give or take a few days for variation, the span of time between the twelfth and sixteenth day (counting day one as the first day of menstrual flow) should encompass the time of ovulation. The sperm live forty-eight hours, so by avoiding these four days and allowing a little leeway, theoretically, one could avoid pregnancy. The trouble is women just aren't that regular.

By taking advantage of instances where known isolated episodes of intercourse have occurred, it has been established that some women have gotten pregnant from intercourse either a few days before their period or a few days after their period, and there is a sneaking suspicion that a woman can even get pregnant during her period. Using the rhythm method helps to cut down on the number of pregnancies, but used alone it's not the most desirable form of birth control. If the goal is to prevent pregnancies, there are some other things which can be done to improve the use of the rhythm system.

Dear Dr. Lamb—I was glad to hear you recommend the use of temperatures to help with birth control. In these times when so many people are pushing birth control, it seems strange that this very effective method is going almost completely ignored by many. There are studies showing that this method is more effective than artificial and chemical methods, and on the same order of effectiveness as the pill and intrauterine devices (IUD). As one who uses "temperature rhythm" I can only say it has been a very real asset to my marriage. This method puts the responsibility and control on both husband and wife, and thus gives each a deeper sense of responsibility. I wish more doctors would open their minds to this knowledge.

Comment—This couple has apparently been very satisfied with the use of oral temperature as an adjunct to using the rhythm method. Not everybody would agree with the writer's enthusiastic comments. For example, in response to a column I wrote advising people to use the oral temperature method to help improve the rhythm method, I received the following remarks from a practicing obstetrician:

Dear Dr. Lamb—To state that abstinence at the critical period is safe from a health point of view is limiting the statement to physical health and completely disregards the presence of mental health.

As a practicing gynecologist, I can state that rhythm, for many reasons, for most patients does not work, and in the meanwhile can be devastating to their mental health and actually ruin some marriages and many lives.

Why promulgate the myth of effective contraception via rhythm on the unknowing public and start these brides on their honeymoon with a thermometer in one hand and a "hands off" sign in the other? Certainly once these women become mothers they abandon this method.

Comment—These opposite points of view concern the use of body temperature to pinpoint the actual time of ovulation. It is true that if you take the body temperature each morning before the woman gets out of bed, smokes a cigarette, or engages in any other activity that will affect her metabolism markedly beyond her sleeping state, you can plot these (in tenths of degree) and pretty well tell when ovulation occurs. With the menstrual period the temperature tends to drop steadily until it reaches the point of ovulation, at which point it rises sharply about 0.8 of a degree and then maintains a plateau level until the next menstrual period. However, there are many other things which can affect the body temperature, including a simple respiratory infection.

When the sharp rise occurs in the temperature, ovulation has already occurred, and if the couple had intercourse the preceding day, live sperm may already be in the womb since sperm may live as long as forty-eight hours. While it's not ideal, it does help some couples to more clearly identify the ovulatory period. Some individuals, because of religious and moral beliefs, must use the rhythm system. While this may cause some psychic stress it must be balanced against the psychic stress a person experiences who does something he thinks is morally wrong. There isn't any ideal solution. It would be better if some more effective ways could be developed to pinpoint more accurately the time of ovulation, and work along those lines is being done.

Dr. Albert B. Lorinoz, in California, has tested a method based on the saliva developed by Raymond O. Foster and William F. Busse. There is an enzyme in saliva that is markedly increased at the time of ovulation. A simple paper strip which reacts to chemicals will turn blue when treated with the saliva of a woman who is ovulating. Unlike the temperature graph, the change in enzyme content in the saliva occurs early enough to give a person a forty-eight to seventy-two-hour warning before the onset of ovulation. This is important in any method based on identifying the time of ovulation. This test is not yet available to the public at this writing. It still needs further evaluation and approval of the U.S. Food and Drug Administration. It also offers some other advantages. Some individuals would like to know when ovulation occurs so they can concentrate on inducing a pregnancy by having sexual intercourse at that time.

Another method of determining the time of ovulation is observing the change in the mucus from the cervix and how it affects the vagina. This method too has not yet been subjected to rigorous examination. There is an increased outpouring of mucus or material which resembles raw egg white about two days before ovulation. Actually a woman begins to have an increased amount of wetness of the vaginal area shortly after her menstrual period. This increases in amount and in the two days just before ovulation it reaches its peak. At that point the mucus is clear and slippery. After ovulation the mucus changes and becomes more cloudy and sticky, gradually becoming heavier. The clear, slippery mucus is nature's way of preparing the woman for sexual activity for pregnancy. By avoiding sexual intercourse during this peak of clear mucus secretion and for four days afterwards, it is felt that a woman can improve her chances of avoiding pregnancy. I would not like, at this time, however, to endorse this method as a satisfactory means of birth control, but perhaps the combination of temperature graph, the saliva test, and these observations would improve the use of the rhythm method for those who feel they must use this type of birth control.

THE PILL

Widespread confusion persists about the safety of the pill and what to expect when it is being used. This problem is complicated by the large number of different pills that are available and the many new contraceptive pills that are steadily arriving on the market. To understand the principle of the birth control pill, it is necessary to understand the interaction and sequence of female hormones. There are four principal hormones responsible for the menstrual cycle. Two of these are from the pituitary gland just underneath the brain and the other two are produced by the ovaries. The menstrual cycle is actually controlled by the brain, which in turn controls the time of secreting the hormones to cause ovulation. The two hormones from the pituitary gland stimulate the ovaries to produce the ovarian hormones. If the ovaries quit producing enough hormones, then the pituitary gland pours out more of its stimulating hormones to whip the ovaries into activity. Thus there is a balance between the hormones produced by the pituitary and those produced by the ovaries.

The first important hormone in this scheme is called the follicle-stimulating hormone (FSH). It stimulates the development of the egg in the ovary. As the egg develops like a cyst formation under the influence of FSH, the ovary begins to pour out its first important hormone, estrogen. This hormone is responsible for much of the feminine behavior associated with the menstrual cycle. The word "estrogen" refers to estrus (the mating period) which in Greek and Latin meant gadfly or frenzy. In mammals, as the amount of estrogen increases, the female's sexual desire is increased. It also causes retention of salt and water. About midway in the cycle when the blisterlike follicle is fully ripened and ready to burst, the pituitary stops producing FSH. The increased level of estrogen apparently signals the pituitary that the egg is ready to hatch. Abruptly the gland shifts gears and releases its second hormone, called the lutinizing hormone (LH). This is the hormone that stimulates the actual bursting or hatching of the follicle, or ovulation. When this occurs, there is a sudden, momentary drop in the amount of estrogen produced by the ovary. The second pituitary factor, LH, also stimulates the ruptured blisterlike follicle to form a new structure, called the corpus luteum. It is a small, yellowish body that is chiefly responsible for producing the second ovarian hormone, called progesterone. This ovarian hormone quiets the uterus and helps prepare it for the implantation and growth of the fertilized ovum.

As long as the ovary is producing enough estrogen or progesterone, the pituitary will not form the FSH factor responsible for stimulating follicles and causing ovulation. The principle of birth control pills is to provide enough estrogen and progesterone or varied combinations of these hormones to inhibit the pituitary gland from forming FSH, thereby blocking the ovary from developing mature follicles, and preventing ovulation.

If the egg is not fertilized, pregnancy does not follow and the corpus luteum body degenerates, causing the production of estrogen and progesterone to fall sharply. This drop in female hormones induces the menstrual cycle or shedding of the lining of the uterus. To duplicate the menstrual cycle, the birth control pills are usually stopped after being given for twenty or twenty-one days. Two or three days later, after the withdrawal of female hormone, menstruation starts. The period usually lasts about five days, the woman is off the pill about seven days, and then resumes the cycle again.

The complexities of the pill and its complications are a stimulus for a constant source of letters.

Dear Dr. Lamb—I am fourteen years old and I am on the birth control pill. There are some things I don't understand. I have been on the pill for two months. When I went to get them, I was told that if I had sexual contact with a boy I should use that foam stuff and the boy should use a rubber. Do I have to use that foam, and does the boy have to use the rubber? Will I get pregnant if I or the boy don't use them? I've never had sex with a boy before. Will it hurt bad? Please hurry with an answer.

Comment—The birth control pills are quite effective in preventing pregnancies, but they do not protect against venereal disease. Because the pill affects the normal acidity of the vagina, a girl is more susceptible to gonorrhea while she is on the pill. The foams have not proved to be very successful as a contraceptive or in protecting against disease. The old-fashioned condom, however, is reasonably effective in protecting against venereal disease. If the boy wears a condom, or skin, the mechanical barrier will help protect him from venereal disease should the woman have this problem and it will protect the woman if he should be infected. Otherwise, I see no use for adding these devices to the sexual routine for a person who is taking the pill. With the present epidemic of venereal disease, the advantages of the condom should not be overlooked.

Dear Dr. Lamb—Would you clarify some facts about the pill. I have heard that this method of birth control is not 100 percent sure. Can I become pregnant although I am on a prescribed birth control pill through some malfunction of its ingredients?

Comment—The trick with birth control pills is to provide enough female hormone to inhibit ovulation, and at the same time not give so much as to produce undesirable side effects. Since the side effects limit how much can be given, it's not too surprising that the pills are not 100 percent effective. In the 1969 U.S. Food and Drug Administration's report, oral contraceptives were said to limit pregnancies to about one in 100 women in a year's time. So, literally, your chance is about one in 100 of getting pregnant in a year's time if you're taking the pill. There are differences in pills. Some new preparations use less female hormone, and they are not as effective in preventing pregnancy. Any new pill needs to be tested for a period of time to find out its degree of effectiveness.

Dear Dr. Lamb—I am getting married soon, but don't want children right away. I would like my wife to take birth control pills but I'm worried about their possible adverse side effects. Obviously, anything which affects the bodily processes unnaturally (as does the pill) can't do any good, but what I want to know is how bad is it? Could you briefly advise me as to the facts or alleged facts in this case?

Comment—Perhaps the one side effect that has scared women the most is the possibility of the formation of blood clots which in turn can go to the lungs or brain and even cause death. Other complications have been mentioned which I'll discuss in connection with letters about these problems. The blood clot question still has not been completely resolved. The American Medical Association and the American College of Obstetricians and Gynecologists, in conjunction with the U.S. Food and Drug Administration, estimated that one woman in 2,000 on the pill in a year's time would have a blood clot. Women not on the pill also have blood clots. According to their report for women under thirty-five the death rate from blood clots is one in 66,000 in women on the pill and only one in 500,000 in women not taking the pill. Over thirty-five the death rate is one in 25,000 for pill users and one in 200,000 for nonusers.

The concern about the formation of blood clots has prompted doctors to believe that women who have had histories of clots in the legs, or any other indications of clots in the body, should not use the pill. This question is not completely settled, though, and a recent research report by Dr. Victor Drill and David W. Calhoun of the University of Illinois College of Medicine states that the pill does not increase blood clot formation. Their report has been published in the *Journal of the American Medical Association* which connotes some degree of acceptance. These researchers pointed out that the past studies have all been done as a retrospective study (that means looking back at case histories and trying to see by hindsight what happened to women who were taking the pill). They planned a research study looking forward; that is, they selected their groups of patients for the population to be studied and followed them over a period of time. This method is considered more accurate in research. Their study showed that the incidence of clots in women on the pill was less than one in 1,000 in a year's time, which compares very favorably with the normal incidence in women of childbearing age which is 2.2 cases per 1,000 women in a year's time. In fact the study might make you wonder if the contraceptive pills didn't actually protect against blood clot formation. This study is consistent with an earlier report from the Mayo Clinic which also failed to show that the pill increased blood clots in healthy women.

No doubt this problem will be argued for some time to come, and there will be additional research studies to confirm or refute these points of view. In any case, the likelihood of having a complication of this type caused by the pill is relatively small. It is considerably less than the dangers of a normal pregnancy, including the incidence of blood clots and strokes that occur during the nine-month pregnancy in women.

Dear Dr. Lamb—Can oral contraceptives cause nervousness and depression?

Comment—There have been many reports that they do. However, most studies suggest that this is more apt to occur in women who already have these basic problems. Some women who have been said to have depressive and nervous episodes because of the pill would have had them anyway, and because they're on the pill, it gets the blame.

Dear Dr. Lamb—I started taking birth control pills about seven years ago. After about the second month, I quit having a climax and seemed to lose all my libido. I have gone through all the pills (six or seven kinds) and all had side effects (bleeding, numbness, etc.). I finally quit them altogether about three years ago. I have put on thirty pounds of weight and cannot seem to get it off. I have not had a climax in all that seven years. This is the opposite of what had been before.

Comment—There are a number of women who have reported a decrease in libido and problems with reaching a climax after they started taking the pill. Apparently it does affect some women this way. It's difficult to be certain that this is the cause, though, because there are so many factors which can produce this same effect. In other words, a woman's loss of interest in sex and ability to have a climax may have been caused by some factor other than the pill, including psychological factors.

The problem of weight gain is real. Most of it isn't actual fat, though, it's the retention of salt and water which normally occurs as the result of female hormones. A woman who is unhappy and is not having a satisfactory sex life frequently will eat to compensate for her emotional problems. Excessive eating, regardless of the cause, eventually leads to genuine obesity.

Dear Dr. Lamb—My problem is what is commonly known as "mother's mask." I developed this condition of the face while I was taking the pill. It is far more pronounced after I have spent some time in the sun, while in the winter it is barely noticeable. I quit taking the pill one year ago, but this summer the marks are very bad. I might mention I had this problem with my fourth daughter who was born several months ago, but the marks were gone by the time I left the hospital.

I took the pill for three and a half years and each summer the markings got worse. I want to know if this brownness will ever disappear. Is there something I can do or take to rid myself of this? I love the sun and all activities that go along with summer weather. I would hate to spend my summer indoors.

Comment—This is one of the complications of birth control pills. They do increase the tendency to develop pigmentation in the cheeks and face to produce the so-called mask-of-pregnancy effect. The increased pigmentation during pregnancy is a complication resulting from an increase in the hormones present; therefore, it isn't too surprising that it occurs in a number of women on the pill. Women who have this problem either have to forego the pill or forego the sun, or have brown spots. There is some tendency for the excess pigmentation to disappear in time. If it's already present, one approach is to use sun screen over the area of the pigmentation before exposing one's face to the sun; this helps to even out the browning. Most measures to solve this problem are less than satisfactory.

Dear Dr. Lamb—Four years ago I had a child. I took birth control pills for two years after that. Now for the past two years I have not taken the pill, as I would like to have another baby. So far, I haven't become pregnant. I understand some women do not ovulate again for several years, and in some cases never, after having taken the pill. If this is true, can anything be done to correct it? Also, since being off the pill my menstrual periods have been very irregular. Is this something which will correct itself?

Comment—Both of these observations are accurate. I receive a large number of letters from women who have been on the pill, and who subsequently have trouble getting pregnant. Most doctors say that this problem will persist for no more than six months after a woman has stopped the pill. The large volume of mail I receive on this problem from women who have had this difficulty for a year or more without being able to get pregnant suggests that the time lag is considerably longer. Women with these problems frequently need help to regain their fertility. This includes the administrations of hormones and sometimes fertility pills.

When the pill first came out there was considerable speculation that there would be a rebound fertility period, that when a woman came off the pill, whammo! she would get pregnant immediately. This has not proved to be the case. Some women who can't get pregnant after the pill would have had the problem anyway. About 15 percent of couples have sterility problems.

Dear Dr. Lamb—I'm twenty years old and have migraine headaches. My mother, grandmother, and great-grandmother also had migraines. I take birth control pills, and these seem to increase the frequency of the headaches. Is it dangerous to continue the pill in this situation?

Comment—It depends upon how severely incapacitating the headaches are. It is true that the birth control pills can aggravate migraine headaches in people who are afflicted with this disorder.

Dear Dr. Lamb—During my first month of pregnancy I was still taking birth control pills. Now I am three months pregnant and would like to know if the pills will affect the baby in any way.

Comment—There are no good studies on this, but it is advised that women should not take birth control pills during pregnancy. Accordingly, if a woman is on the pill and she misses two successive cycles, she should go immediately to her doctor to be checked for pregnancy. If she proves to be pregnant, she should stop taking the pill. It is unlikely that the pill will seriously affect the baby during the first two-cycle phase.

Dear Dr. Lamb—I am seventeen and taking birth control pills which I got from a doctor. I am confused and do not know whether or not I should continue taking them, because I heard they can cause breast cancer. Is this true? If I continue to take them for five years straight and then wish to have a baby, will this cause the baby to be born deformed?

Comment—There is no proof that birth control pills cause cancer. This problem has been investigated, and there is no hard evidence that it increases this likelihood. It is true that a person who already has cancer, for example, a breast cancer, should not take the birth control pills. There is no evidence that subsequent pregnancies after having gone off the pill will be associated with birth defects.

Dear Dr. Lamb—I am fifty and have been a widow for six and a half years, but I am to be married again in six weeks. Because of my age I do not want to have children and would like to use birth control pills, but my doctor refused to give me a prescription. He said it was not wise for a woman of my age to go on the pill for the first time. It is true that I have never used them previously. I talked to my gynecologist and he gave me a prescription, saying he thought it would be good for me since my menopause would be prolonged. He saw no danger in my taking the pills. I would like to have the freedom of the pills but I do not want it bad enough to take a dangerous chance. What should I do?

Comment—There isn't any reason that a fifty-year-old woman should not take birth control pills unless she has one of the recognized medical contraindications, like blood clots or cancer. In fact, since they are composed of female hormones, they are often used to maintain the recurrent menstrual cycle or to delay the effects of the menopause. Some women continue to take them for years after the time of the natural menopause for just that purpose.

CREAMS AND FOAMS

The idea of putting something in the vagina to either act as a barrier against the sperm or kill the sperm is not exactly new. The oldest record of a spermicide was that used by the Egyptians in 1850 B.C. They used crocodile dung in a paste-like mixture. Human imagination hasn't left much out since then. These agents work to change the acidity of the female vagina. However, the vagina is already acid and will kill the sperm within six to eight hours. The sperm that survive the normal forty-eight-hour period are those that have penetrated the cervical barrier and have entered the womb, far beyond the acid environment of the vagina. Judging from the number of letters received, only a small number of people use foams or creams as a birth control procedure.

Dear Dr. Lamb—We are a young married couple and we don't plan to have children right away. Just lately we tried a foam about one week after my wife's period. Since then we had a party with just our close friends and talked about sex and contraceptives. Someone said they used this foam and still nine months later there was Junior. My wife and I followed the directions carefully, but we are still wondering if the foam is any good or if it isn't. Could you tell us something about the foam? We don't want to use pills because of all the wrong happenings they cause.

Comment—The foams are thought to be slightly better than the creams or jellies, but neither one is outstanding as an agent in preventing pregnancy. According to the U.S. Food and Drug Administration's report of 1969, individuals who use vaginal foam can expect to have 28.3 pregnancies in 100 women over a year's time, and those who use the jelly or cream alone can expect a rate of 36.8 pregnancies per 100 women over a year's time. This is better than using no contraception though, which yields a pregnancy rate of 80 out of 100 women in the course of a year. In brief, don't expect too much from the foam and jelly contraceptives.

INTRAUTERINE DEVICES (IUD)

There appears to be a steady growth in acceptance of these devices. Also there are continued refinements which make them more effective than the earlier models. The intrauterine devices, literally, are objects that have been placed in the uterus to prevent pregnancy. The idea is not new, even ancient camel drivers were known to put stones in the uterus of their camels to prevent them from getting pregnant on long treks. There are a number of different devices including loops, spirals, T's, and shields. More recent devices have been shaped to fit the uterus better than some of the earlier ones and are less likely to be expelled. Some of them use copper which is also thought to help prevent pregnancy.

Not all women have been happy with IUD's. They do increase menstrual bleeding and sometimes cause mid-menstrual spotting. The midpoint of the menstrual cycle is the

92

time when the uterus is most susceptible to bleeding, and with an IUD in place there is more likelihood that this will occur. In general, women who are using the IUD should have more frequent checks on their blood count and will need to pay more attention to their diet to be certain they get enough iron or else actually take iron supplement pills regularly. A few women have complained of cramps and discomfort with the IUD when it is first in place. Some of the new devices may minimize some of the earlier problems that have been experienced with the IUD. Despite some problems with the earlier models, it appears to be a good and effective means of birth control.

Dear Dr. Lamb—I have some questions about intrauterine devices. Can a woman who has been fitted with such a device by her doctor become pregnant if the device stays in place and causes her no other problems? If a woman does become pregnant while she has the coil still in place, will its presence harm her baby or will it have to be removed? If it is removed early in the pregnancy, will the fetus be unharmed and the pregnancy go along normally?

Comment—Yes, women do get pregnant while they have the device in place. The U.S. Food and Drug Administration's report of 1969 rates IUD's with a pregnancy incidence of less than 3 in 100 women over a year's time. Some of the newer devices claim a 99.5 percent effectiveness. If a woman does get pregnant, the baby can develop normally with the device in place, and it is delivered on the surface of the membranes at the time of birth. The baby is not delivered clutching the intrauterine device in its hand as has been reported for amusement. It is usually not necessary to remove the device. If it were removed successfully early, the pregnancy could proceed normally.

Dear Dr. Lamb—I am a mother of four children, and I am twenty-five years old. About three months ago my doctor inserted an IUD to protect me from pregnancy.

He said it would work for about a year, after which I would have to go back to have it changed. A friend of mine told me that the IUD will cause me to have cancer. Is that right? I am worried about this, and I'm thinking about going back to my doctor to have it taken out.

Comment—There is absolutely no evidence that the IUD causes cancer in women, although from the number of letters I have received on the subject it seems to be a common fear. This is a wild rumor without basis of fact.

Dear Dr. Lamb—Regarding the IUD, my doctor said it should be replaced within two years because they become crusted. I had always thought the same one could be worn indefinitely. When mine was inserted the string stayed curled up next to the device. Therefore, I don't have any string and I would have to have a D&C to have it removed. Would this removal really be necessary?

Comment—Doctors' opinions vary about how soon an IUD should be replaced. Some doctors leave them in for five years or more.

DIAPHRAGMS

There was a time when the diaphragm was the kingpin of birth control. This was before the days of pills and before the IUD became acceptable. The diaphragm was thought to be a mechanical barrier to the sperm. A jellylike substance was placed over the cervix, theoretically to help kill the sperm. The diaphragm method of birth control is not nearly as effective as tubal ligation, the pill, or IUD. According to the U.S. Food and Drug Administration's 1969 report, the diaphragm with the jelly still permitted approximately 18 pregnancies in 100 women in a year's time. The relative unreliability of the diaphragm can be clearly understood on the basis of Masters and Johnson's work. They showed that during sexual activity, the size of the vaginal barrel widens and

94

elongates. Even the best-fitting diaphragm moves freely during intercourse. Thus the rubber diaphragm does not provide a mechanical barrier to sperm, and the effectiveness of the procedure rests primarily in the barrier caused by the jelly blocking the cervical entrance.

WITHDRAWAL TECHNIQUE

Many people still rely on the withdrawal technique as a means of preventing pregnancies. It was found to be one of the most frequent methods used by college girls having an active sexual life. On this method, the man withdraws from the vagina just before he reaches an orgasm, thereby avoiding spilling any of the semen in the vaginal cavity. Many authorities have felt that this has a bad psychological effect because it does not adequately relieve the sexual tensions of the couple. Actually a well-conditioned male can bring a responsive partner to climax before he reaches orgasm. Since it is quite possible for both partners to reach an orgasm by this method, the common criticism that it induces psychic tensions is not well supported by the facts. The greatest risk is that a small amount of semen will escape before the penis is withdrawn, and it is these first few drops that contain the most sperm cells. It is well to remember that even a small amount of sperm spilled near the vaginal opening could migrate into the vagina and induce a pregnancy.

Dear Dr. Lamb—Several days ago you wrote on the side effects of the pill. I want you to meet my good friend, Onan, whom I met in the 38th chapter of Genesis. He has a bad name and the Lord killed him, not for his deed but for his motive. Onan invented or discovered the perfect pill, and I used it with perfect success and real satisfaction for many years. I have two fine sons now happily married for whom I did not plan. My wife just asked me to leave the semen in. There are no side effects and no expense and no loss of pleasure.

Comment—The Bible does refer to this method of birth control and it's sometimes misinterpreted to read that the passage refers to masturbation, which it does not. Onan spilled his seeds on the ground, not from masturbation, but from use of the withdrawal technique. This reader's letter indicates that he has achieved complete satisfaction through the years with this means of birth control. It is not always reliable in terms of preventing pregnancy, although it's in about the same ballpark as the use of the diaphragm. The rate of pregnancy between couples practicing the withdrawal technique is approximately 18 in 100 women over a year's time.

ABORTION

A 1972 United Nations report revealed that abortion may be the most common form of birth control in the world. There are more abortions than babies in eastern Europe where the attitude toward abortions is relatively liberal. In Poland, Czechoslovakia, Yugoslavia, and Hungary, there are over 130 abortions for every 100 live births. The UN study stated that the procedure was relatively safe as compared to the death rate and complications from normal pregnancy. For example, in 100,000 abortions the deaths were as follows: 1.2 in Hungary, 2.5 in Czechoslovakia, 4.1 in Japan, 4.5 in Yugoslavia, 39 in Sweden and 41 in Denmark.

The reason for the increased mortality in Sweden and Denmark was attributed to the fact that they permit abortions after the initial three months of pregnancy. The mortality risk of an abortion increases sharply as the pregnancy progresses. The mortality rates for pregnancy are about 20 deaths per 100,000 pregnancies in the more advanced countries, and as high as over 300 in underdeveloped countries. Regardless of one's moral attitude concerning abortions, it seems that they are here to stay. Individuals with different moral attitudes have quite opposite points of view about this problem and feel quite strongly about it.

Dear Dr. Lamb—I am twenty years old and pregnant. The

96

father is the same age and not working. I know the facts of life, but I never thought it would happen to me. My mother and I talked, and she said if anything like that ever happened to me, she didn't want to ever know about it and I agree. I think she deserves better. What I want to know is who do I see for an abortion? I'm scared to go to my doctor because he's my mom's also. Please hurry with your reply. I'm already about a month along.

Comment—This is an all too common story, and it's quite true that everybody seems to think it's going to happen to someone else and not to them. From some letters I have received from the pro abortion group, they would have me recommend that this girl be hustled off to the nearest doctor who would be willing to perform an abortion. Those who are vitally opposed to abortion feel that she should not be permitted to have one. My advice is that despite her reluctance to do so, she should see her family doctor. If she doesn't want to see him because he also takes care of her mother, then she should make a point to visit a new family doctor or go see an obstetrician and gynecologist. She can get the name of a specialist in this area from her county medical society.

Doctors are quite familiar with this problem because of its frequency. Seeing the doctor first has many advantages. First, he can determine whether or not the girl is pregnant. Some girls think they're pregnant when in reality they're not. Second, he can determine whether or not the girl has any serious disease. Considering the frequency of venereal disease in this age, this is an important consideration. Finally, the doctor is apt to be well versed in where abortions are legally available and the complications that may result from one. He will also know about the alternatives—where an unwed mother can go to have her baby. In this case the baby can be given up for adoption if the mother elects to do so.

There are many people who would like to have children and can't. They are eager for available babies for adoption. If the family doctor also takes care of the rest of the family, he may be familiar with the family situation and know whether or not it's advisable to discuss the matter with the parents. In many states a doctor is not obliged to discuss a teen-ager's medical problems with the parents.

I do not agree that it is essential to exclude the parents from this experience in a young girl's life. Although parents don't like to face these problems, as is indicated in this letter, the truth is they also don't wish to abandon their children in their hour of need. One of the important benefits of the family is the support, advice and comfort they can give in periods of stress. An unwanted pregnancy in an unwed young girl is such an occasion.

Dear Dr. Lamb—Recently you gave advice to a fifteen-year-old girl who thought she might be pregnant and wanted to know where she could get counseling. You advised her to see her family doctor, which was fine. You also told her there was a book available where she could find out information about abortions. This was simply an open invitation for her to get one. If doctors refused to murder babies, women would not consider this grizzly and disgusting butchery of the most helpless and innocent.

If life is an accident at conception, then it can also be considered an accident at old age, illness, deformity, and any inconvenient time. All we need to do is legalize murder and then add on amendments to see this horror in our day. This country has thousands of couples seeking babies through adoption which are not available. There is no unwanted child, as someone somewhere always wants one. Doctors perpetuating irresponsibility of women by performing abortions are a disgrace to their profession.

I am still in awe of the magnificent uniqueness of my baby son, and the thought that people take it upon themselves to destroy a human life is abhorrent. There is but one God and he laid down the law, even for doctors.

98

Comment—This letter exemplifies clearly the anti-abortion stance. I do not propose to tell people what their moral beliefs should be, but rather to provide them with information and allow them to be responsible for their own morals. There is certainly room for major disagreements concerning the moral and ethical aspects of abortion. Even such items as the definition of when life actually begins is a debatable point. Does life begin when the baby is born, or does life begin at the exact instant that the sperm cell unites with the ovum? It's not likely that a single opinion is going to resolve these hotly debated issues.

Dear Dr. Lamb—I've been told that if you are pregnant (about a month or two), if you drink a couple of bottles of castor oil it will induce your period, causing you to lose the fertilized egg. I would like to know whether or not this is true, and if it will have any other side effects.

Comment—You can bet it will have some side effects, and anyone trying this procedure should stay close to the bathroom. Most of the products taken to induce abortion are completely ineffective. They have little or no effect upon the pregnancy. The only time that they are successful in inducing an abortion is when they produce such a toxic reaction in the mother that her health is endangered as well. There are many products that have been stated to have this effect, and some are sold in drugstores, not necessarily legally. Fortunately most of them are harmless.

There are new preparations being developed which offer the possibility of inducing abortion early in pregnancy. Some of these have been popularly dubbed as the "morning-after pill." These are still in the experimental state, but there is every reason to believe that in the near future a woman will be able to detect a pregnancy early in its course by simple testing at home and that she will be able to take some form of medication, possibly a hormone, to induce normal menstruation, thereby terminating a pregnancy within its first few weeks.

In the meantime it's sound advice to tell people not to try any do-it-yourself abortions, and not to go to anyone besides a reputable physician for information and guidance on any such procedure. It is very dangerous for women to obtain illegal abortions in many localities. In the interest of protecting women's health, I am forced to state that if a woman absolutely insists on having an abortion, she would be well advised to go to a location where such procedures are legal and where they can be done with proper medical safety. This remark does not constitute a blanket endorsement of abortion, but rather a blanket repudiation of illegal abortion with all its hazards and seaminess.

V

Sterility

HISTORY IS STUDDED with examples of couples wanting a child as an heir to the family fortune or an heir to the throne. Progeny are considered by many the closest thing to immortality. Children are the living proof of the father's potency and the mother's fecundity. As such they symbolize proof of the man's masculinity and woman's femininity. No wonder they are important to the self-image and ego structures of the parents. Within the bedroom communities of the United States many couples' lives revolve around the rearing of the children. The child, his playmates, and social activities become the dominant, overriding factor in the living pattern. There are the school activities of the children, the swimming lessons, the art lessons, Boy Scouts for the boys, Girl Scouts for the girls, parent-teacher association meetings and many opportunities for social interchange of the parents such as Cub Scout leader, Den Mother, and president of the PTA. To be without children in one of these bedroom communities is to be a social outcast and many childless couples feel a sense of social stigma.

In the United States 15 percent of all married couples are sterile. The problem is not unique. A couple is judged to be sterile if they cohabited without use of birth control for a year's time without a pregnancy. Considering the frequency of this problem and the distress it causes the individuals concerned, it is not surprising that many people write to me about their sterility problems.

Dear Dr. Lamb—I will be twenty soon and my problem is that I can't get pregnant. My period is quite irregular, sometimes one and one-half months late, and it ranges from one and one-half days to six days in length, but it usually averages four days. I am overweight, weighing 206½ pounds and am five feet, six inches tall. Will this affect my chances of getting pregnant? My only nervous or bad habit is eating. I seem to do that constantly.

Comment—Whenever a couple is having a sterility problem the first step is a complete medical examination of both partners. There are many medical abnormalities that can contribute to the problem. This includes thyroid function as well as other types of endocrine disorders which may not be directly associated with the sexual organs. Correction of any underlying medical problem has often solved the problem.

Some couples have trouble getting pregnant because basically they lack necessary information about sex. To illustrate this problem, there are rare case reports of women who go to the doctor's office complaining of sterility and have an intact hymen membrane. This occurs in rare cases when the female urethral tube has been distended enough to be used as a sexual organ. Dr. Albert Altchek, obstetrician and gynecologist, states this can occur in congenital absence of the vagina or simple vaginal stenosis. The woman can be stimulated sexually this way to orgasm since the clitoris and surrounding tissues receive mechanical stimulation even though the wrong opening is used. This is only one example of problems people can have with the simple sex act.

It is important that the precise sexual habits of the couple be reviewed. Some women who have problems with fertility are found to be using foams designed to kill sperm for lubricants. Others jump out of bed at the instant of ejaculation and rush to the bathroom to clean up rather than resting comfortably to give the sperm cells in the pool of semen lying at the mouth of the cervix an opportunity to enter the uterus, migrate to the tube and initiate pregnancy.

Other couples are totally unaware of the necessity for relatively frequent intercourse to achieve pregnancy. While once or twice a year might cause a pregnancy, the chances are greatly reduced. Other couples are not well informed about the menstrual cycle and do not appreciate when the most fertile time actually occurs. The same information used for birth control can be applied to induce pregnancy. In women who are regular the fertile period is at the midpoint between menstrual cycles, or approximately fourteen days before the onset of menstruation.

Women can pinpoint the time of ovulation by using the oral temperature technique that is also used for birth control. By taking the temperature daily before getting out of bed or doing anything else that might speed up the body's activities and plotting it in tenths of degrees, the sudden change in temperature at the time of ovulation can be determined. The ovum only survives about six to eight hours, while the sperm cells can live about forty-eight hours under normal conditions. When it is determined that ovulation has occurred there is no time to waste.

A change in the woman's secretions is also an indication of ovulation. The increased amount and the thinning and clearing of the mucus are indicative that the time of ovulation is near. Saliva tests, or other procedures which may eventually become available, that help pinpoint the time of ovulation can also be useful in helping to take advantage of the opportune time to induce pregnancy.

Dear Dr. Lamb—I am twenty-three years old and I stopped my period four months after I got married four years ago, and I haven't had but three since then. My husband and I want a baby very badly. Can one get pregnant without a period? Is there anything I can do about this that I don't know about? I have been going to the doctor for three years.

Comment—Clearly this woman has a fertility problem. Within three years time a doctor should certainly be able to judge whether a woman is truly infertile or not. Within this length of time he should also have learned whether it would be useful to try some of the fertility pills or other methods which might improve the chances of pregnancy.

The absence of a menstrual period does not prove that ovulation does not occur. The presence or absence of ovulation can be determined by the temperature chart that I have mentioned before. The question of adequacy of female hormones and the response of the uterus can be determined by taking a small piece of tissue from the lining of the body of the uterus and examining it under a microscope. This is an important test in evaluating a woman for a sterility problem.

Not all problems of infertility can be solved. In fact only a relatively small portion of the couples who have sterility problems can be helped to have a child, if there is truly some medical problem. In most studies, a little over a third of the sterility problems are caused by the male. Some of these can be corrected and some cannot. Only about 15 percent of the sterility problems are caused by hormone factors and only part of these can be corrected by administering various hormonal preparations.

One of the important examinations that should be performed is a vaginal examination very shortly after intercourse. This is very helpful in determining how long the sperm lives in the vaginal vault, as well as other factors which may contribute to the problem of sterility. But just as a woman may get pregnant in her later years whether or not she is having a period, the same thing can happen to a woman at any age. It is a mistake to assume that just because the woman isn't menstruating she can't get pregnant.

Dear Dr. Lamb—I am twenty years old and have been married for almost two years. I have never used any type of birth control, yet I have not become pregnant. My question is, can too much sex be the cause of my problem? My husband and I have had sex every night. Sometimes twice. Twice I thought I was pregnant because I missed my period for almost three months, but apparently I wasn't. My periods are sometimes irregular. Could this have anything to do with the problem?

I have never consulted a doctor on this so I don't know whether it is physical.

Comment—As in all such cases, a doctor's examination is the first step. There are a number of individuals who think that too much sex can cause infertility. There is no evidence that this is really true in normal, healthy, sexually active people. There are a few disorders in which this can become a factor. If the man's sperm count is relatively low, it is sometimes best for him to expend his efforts at or near the time of ovulation. In other words, the man saves his ammunition until the target is in sight, but abstaining from sex for more than three to five days will not help with this problem. Having sexual relations every night is not particularly unusual and most often is conducive to pregnancy, unless there are some other difficulties.

Menstrual irregularities are quite common. Sometimes they are an indication of an underlying hormone problem which might need correcting. In other instances it is an indication of a problem with the uterus (womb), and during examination the physician may elect to do a dilatation and curettage (D&C). This calls for dilating the cervix and scraping of the lining of the uterus, thus giving it a chance to develop new tissues. This sometimes is very helpful in adjusting matters to a more normal routine and can result in a subsequent pregnancy.

Dear Dr. Lamb—Could a number of x-ray pictures (about six) taken on the upper part of the back cause a woman to be sterile?

Comment—Not likely. It is true that excess radiation can cause sterility but this is much more likely to happen in the male than in the female, because the testicles are exposed outside of the body cavity. X-ray, like heat, has to penetrate an object to produce an effect internally. Six ordinary X-rays are not unusual, and should have no effect.

Dear Dr. Lamb—I am having a problem with getting pregnant. I have a girl friend who has had the same problem and after all of her examinations and medicine she still didn't get pregnant. Her doctor said something like her body is supposed to be fighting her husband's sperm by attacking and destroying them. I wonder if my body could be doing this too?

Comment—This is possible. There is no one simple answer to the problem of sterility since there are so many factors that can be involved. If it is demonstrated that the woman ovulates regularly and her entire female system is in good order and that the man also is in good order, then it is worthwhile looking into this possibility. In such cases the woman develops an immune reaction to the sperm cells just as we develop an immune reaction to various infectious agents; thus, when the foreign agent or sperm is introduced into the body, the woman's chemical immunity acts to destroy or kill the sperm. There are certain sophisticated tests which can be done to demonstrate this.

People lose immunity to diseases as years go by if they are not exposed to the disease again. This is why smallpox shots have to be repeated and a number of other vaccinations have to be repeated or "booster shots" are given. A person can take advantage of this principle by removing the stimulus to the antibodies against sperm—this means preventing the woman's body from coming in contact with semen or sperm. The two chief ways of doing this are to abstain from intercourse altogether, which is not very practical in married life, or to use a condom. By trapping the semen in the condom and making sure that none of it gets in the woman's vagina eventually her immunity or resistance to the sperm will diminish. A good working program would be to use the condom for sexual relations for a period of six months and then stop using it. In a fairly large sample of couples who have tried this, approximately half subsequently had pregnancies.

Dear Dr. Lamb—I was recently told that I could never have children. I am in my early twenties and this is very depressing. My tubes are blocked or grown together. My doctor doesn't know exactly what it is, but the dye he injected wouldn't go inside my tubes. There is an operation I could have but my doctor doesn't recommend it because most of them haven't been successful. We have heard of several cases where it has been successful and some where it hasn't. I am undecided on what to do.

Comment—Blocked tubes is one of the common causes of sterility in the female. This and other anatomical defects that function as a natural block between the ovum and the sperm account for over one third of the problems of sterility. There are a large number of inflamatory or infectious diseases that can cause this. One cause is gonorrhea, although I hasten to add that there are many other kinds of inflammation that can also cause this difficulty. Having blocked tubes does not mean the woman has had gonorrhea. In some instances the tubes appear to have been blocked throughout life.

If it can accurately be established that the tubes have been blocked, and depending on the nature of the block and what has to be done to achieve a repair, a surgical procedure can be attempted. Such surgical procedures are of no value in a woman who is not ovulating or has other factors which cause or contribute to her sterility. Nor are they of any value to the woman if the husband is sterile, unless she chooses to consider artificial insemination or obtaining a new partner.

There is great diversity in the reported successes of operations to open the tubes. It is fair to say that in ordinary types of surgical procedures, the success rate may be as low as one out of four. Nevertheless even that low rate offers a chance for the sterile couple when there are no complications. A blocked tube prevents the ovum from passing down the tube and the sperm from passing up the tube. Thus, they never meet and pregnancy does not occur. Techniques are constantly being perfected to correct the block. Recently, Dr. Celso-Raymon Garcia at the University of Pennsylvania has developed a microsurgery technique. By using a microscope it is easier to see the delicate structures and hopefully repair them. He has reported that the operation has been successful in opening the tubes in about half of his cases and that some of these women have subsequently had successful pregnancies. This same type of operation is used to repair tubes that have been tied as a birth control measure for women who have wished to reverse the procedure in hopes of having another pregnancy.

Dear Dr. Lamb—My husband and I have been married seven years and we have no children. The problem is that I only ovulate on the average of once a year. This has been determined by charting my temperature and by studying the tissue from my womb (endometrial biopsy). I took Clomid for five days and about twelve days later I ovulated. I have not taken it since. Please tell me what the chances are of my having a multiple birth using Clomid.

Comment—There are some new products now available which stimulate the ovary and can cause a small percentage of women with sterility problems to become pregnant. These are the women, like this letter writer, who do not ovulate. The ovaries are perfectly normal and there is an ample supply of egg cells but the stimulus from the pituitary gland to release the egg is missing or faulty. These new medicines stimulate the ovary to normal function so that ovulation occurs and pregnancy is possible. Basically then, these products replace the normal function of one of the hormones from the pituitary gland underneath the brain.

Clomid is one of the fertility drugs that has this effect.

In a report from the Medical College of Georgia on 800 women using Clomid, less than 9 percent had twins and there were no incidences of triplets. Some of the fertility pills that have been used have stimulated the ovaries to mature more than one egg at a time. The dosage is also a factor. These have been responsible for the recent rash of multiple births, triplets, quads and quintuplets.

It is often necessary to give other hormones at the end of the five-day period to induce ovulation. For women whose problem is limited to a simple failure to ovulate because of inadequate stimulation from a pituitary hormone, these new medicines offer considerable hope of a successful pregnancy. They will not, of course, correct problems of obstructed tubes, difficulties caused by the male partner, or faulty techniques in intercourse, including the use of lubricants that kill sperm.

Dear Dr. Lamb—My husband and I would like to have another baby but my doctor does not believe I am ovulating and would like to give me a small amount of fertility pills to stimulate my ovaries. Can you tell me what the risks are to me and to the baby I would conceive? My primary concern is that the egg I produced might not be normal because of the artificial stimulation.

Comment—The likelihood of having an abnormal child because of fertility stimulation is relatively remote. The biggest problem to occur has been the increased possibility of multiple births with premature delivery. These cause the same problems as any premature birth: if the babies are too small or too premature they may not have developed enough to survive.

Dear Dr. Lamb—If a woman is taking a fertility pill to bring about ovulation, would it be possible for her to conceive and give birth to twins with separate fathers if she is having an affair and having relations also with her husband?

Comment—Everything is possible. There was a news account of a case in Germany of a woman who had twins and it was determined by the courts that the twins had different fathers. This could occur if a woman released two eggs and within a short time span had intercourse with two different men. Since sperm cells can survive as long as forty-eight hours, if sperm cells from both men are in the tube, a cell from each of the different men could unite with one egg. As a result the woman could have twins from two different fathers. The way to prevent this problem is obvious.

Dear Dr. Lamb—In a recent article you mentioned that seminal fluid can be examined under a microscope to determine a sperm count. However, you failed to mention how the doctor takes the semen from the male. I want to be tested for sterility and need to know. Does the doctor inject a needle through the donor's scrotum into the testes or does the donor use his hands to ejaculate the sperm?

Comment—The best way to collect a good semen specimen is for the man to masturbate and collect the semen in a wide-mouthed bottle or appropriate container provided for this purpose. The specimen should then be examined while it is still fresh. As such, the method of getting the specimen is considerably less painful than anything imagined by this reader.

Most doctors ask the man to abstain from sexual activity for a period of three to five days prior to obtaining a specimen. This is to provide an ample opportunity for a maximum number of sperm cells and time to produce a normal specimen.

The actual volume of the specimen should be a little less than a teaspoonful of fluid and this amount of fluid should contain at least 20,000,000 sperm cells and 60 percent of these should be motile or moving around on their own power under the microscope. Usually there are many more than this. Each of the sperm cells has a whiplike tail and is able to move around. This is the way they propel themselves up the womb into the tube and impregnate the ovum.

Dear Dr. Lamb—Will you please tell me if the sperm changes in a man from time to time? If the sperm is on the weak side can anything be done to help increase it? My husband had his checked and it was on the weak side. The doctor gave him some pills to help and he goes back in two months. However, it wasn't until he was home that he wondered about the painting since he had been painting our house. My husband himself said he didn't think the specimen looked right when he took it to the doctor.

Comment—One episode of housepainting is not likely to cause a problem with the man's fertility. It is true that certain occupations expose an individual to increased amounts of metals such as lead and can contribute to sterility. These occupations include painting, plumbing and printing. Men who are overweight, lead sedentary lives, and wear tight underwear are also more likely to have problems. This is true if there is a marginal situation to begin with and less likely to be true for individuals with normal potency.

There is an important distinction between potency and sterility. A man may be relatively sterile and be a first-class sexual athlete. Sexual prowess is no guarantee that the semen will contain large amounts of viable sperm. A good example of this is the man who has a vasectomy and retains his sexual capacity. Of course if a man is impotent or otherwise unable to engage in sexual intercourse then, regardless of how many cells might be in any semen which seeps out, he is not likely to impregnate his wife.

Dear Dr. Lamb—Can a man be sterile for many years and become potent long enough to become a father and then become sterile after that again?

Comment—It sounds like someone is on the hook. It is unlikely that this would occur but it is not impossible. It only takes one sperm cell and one ovum united under the right circumstances to induce a pregnancy.

The inability to produce adequate amounts of sperm cells is frequently caused by atherosclerosis or fatty deposits in the arteries. The testicles are one of the first organs in the body to be affected by this condition. This is the same process that affects the arteries to cause heart attack. The fatty deposits in the arteries diminish the blood supply to the testicles. In the absence of sufficient oxygen and nutrition, the process of forming new sperm cells is significantly curtailed. Sections of male testicles show that the parts responsible for forming sperm cells actually degenerate and the size of the testicles decreases.

Within the body of the testicle there are two types of cells

111

—one produces the sperm which are stored in the tubules until they are gradually moved out into the main tube or vas deferens or finally carried out with the semen during the sex act. The other cells lie between the tubules and are the specialized cells that produce the male hormone or testosterone. As the fatty deposits in the arteries continue in men, eventually the ratio between male and female hormone production is reversed. This is part of the reason that older men sometimes develop significant changes in their voice, and that other feminization characteristics accompany increasing years. This observation of the frequency of atherosclerosis in the testicles and its effect on their function is adequate justification for any man to be concerned about preventing fatty deposits in his arteries, not just to avoid a heart attack but also to maintain his manhood.

Despite the frequency of fatty deposits in the arteries, many men quite advanced in years are found to have active, normal sperm cells. Some of these are observed in the prostate gland during an autopsy. There are quite enough incidents of older men fathering children to substantiate this point. As the production of sperm cells begins to diminish it's possible for a man to have a specimen that is sufficiently low in sperm count to classify him as sterile and still subsequently produce enough live sperm cells to produce a pregnancy.

In a reported study of one man 119 years old, a semen specimen proved that he still maintained adequate amounts of sperm to father a child. He was from the Abkhasian group of people in Russia who are known for their long and active lives, often living to one hundred years of age or more. The areas of the world where older men are said to retain their potency are also the areas of the world where heart disease is less common. Since both are caused by fatty deposits in the arteries, this is logical. A proper diet, an exercise program and abstaining from smoking are all important measures to prevent fatty deposits from forming in arteries.

Dear Dr. Lamb—My husband and I have been married over three years. The problem is we both want a child very badly. My husband has had a sperm count test and the urologist said that it confirms that he had a lowered count but he didn't offer any treatment or cure for this. Can vitamin E be beneficial and if not what would you suggest? Is it possible to improve our chances of pregnancy by my taking the fertility drug?

Comment—There are many reasons why a man's sperm count may be low, including low thyroid function. Vitamin E has been used to successfully treat sterility in rats with a vitamin E deficiency. There is no proof that it is helpful in man since it is almost impossible for a person on a normal diet to have a Vitamin E deficiency. Taken in reasonable amounts (400 units or less a day) Vitamin E can't cause any harm, however, if one wished to use it. In very large doses it might cause difficulties, but these are doses far beyond the level that most people would be using. Vitamin E is not a sexual stimulant for a man and I don't want to encourage people to think that it would be. If the man has a medical problem such as a low thyroid count, administration of thyroid or correction of an underlying medical problem can often improve his sperm count. In other instances improved living habits, including eliminating cigarettes, excess coffee, alcohol, decreasing obesity, and maintaining a regular exercise program, seem to help improve the body's total function and the likelihood of producing semen with adequate amounts of sperm cells.

Fertility drugs are normally given to a woman who has difficulty ovulating. If she is ovulating normally, fertility drugs are not likely to improve her chances of pregnancy. It would be better to concentrate on correcting or improving the situation in the male. If a woman knows exactly when her ovulation occurs it might be wise to abstain from intercourse from three to five days before this period and then take advantage of the time of ovulation. This will provide a semen specimen with the maximum number of healthy sperm cells in it.

Dear Dr. Lamb—In males if they have had the mumps in

113

infancy or after growing up, does it stop them from being productive? I have never heard of this before.

Comment—It depends on what happens. If the mumps involves the testicles it can damage them and sometimes cause them to shrink in size. This is true whether the person is an adult or a child. This is more apt to occur, however, in the young adult male. If the testicles are involved, the chance of sterility depends on how much damage is done. This is only one cause for sterility in the male. It does not necessarily decrease the male's capacity for the sex act or his own enjoyment.

In one large series of men studied for sterility the most common cause for this problem was found to be the presence of a varicocele. This accounted for almost 40 percent of the causes of decreased fertility in men. A varicocele literally is a varicose vein of the testicle, and the large dilated veins will cause a mass in the scrotum near the testicle which is attached to the cord of the testicle. It is often described as feeling like a bag of worms, because of the dilated, tortuous, blood-filled veins.

A varicocele causes decreased fertility by affecting the temperature control mechanism in the testicles. The artery and vein in the cord of the testicle are laid together in such a way that heat is lost from the artery and picked up by the vein. This cools the arterial blood that arrives at the testicle as much as three degrees below the rest of the body temperature. The testicles must be kept relatively cool to produce normal sperm. When the veins are dilated so that the blood isn't drained properly from the testicles they can no longer induce this cooling effect and this affects the formation of sperm. Correction of varicoceles in a number of men improved their fertility.

Dear Dr. Lamb—We have a very happy marriage founded on a deep belief that marriage is a God-given institution. My husband was forty-six when we married and he has two boys. We want so much to have a child but he has had surgery and isn't able to. I am twenty-three and very healthy so we have been considering artificial insemination. We have seen several doctors but we can't find anyone who will treat this subject as if it were not a bad word or a perverted idea. Most doctors won't even tell us where to write for information. Could you tell us what to do?

Comment—It is true that obtaining information about artificial insemination is difficult in many areas. It is a very successful procedure, as has been proved by animal husbandry. The use of artificial insemination in the cattle industry has enabled cattlemen to rapidly improve their breeds. Stated frankly, the cattle industry is far ahead of the medical profession in the application of artificial insemination. Of course the main difference is the attitudes of society and legal factors which vary from state to state, making it impossible to give a definite answer to this question. Perhaps the best source of information is the Department of Obstetrics and Gynecology at the nearest university medical center. If you get an unsatisfactory reply from the center in your own state then try another state which might have different laws. Planned Parenthood-World Population, at 515 Madison Avenue, New York, New York 10023, can also provide the name and location of clinics treating infertility— in this way you could find the best location for possible artificial insemination.

There are many problems in accomplishing artificial insemination and it is technically not always simple since the woman has to be available at the time that she is fertile. This means that the time of ovulation must be accurately pinpointed and sometimes it takes several sessions in order to achieve this successfully.

It is wise not to overlook the other possibilities in a situation such as this lady describes. If the man has had surgery to induce sterility, it can sometimes be corrected by a repair procedure.

Dear Dr. Lamb—My husband and I have been married almost two years and we haven't been able to have any

115

children yet. We have consulted a specialist and found out there is nothing keeping me from conceiving, but my husband has a low sperm count and it is also deficient. Now he accepts the idea that there is nothing that can be done about it. My husband is taking some kind of hormone pills every morning, and he has had two tests and his sperm is still low and deficient. What I want to know is, is there anything that can be done to improve the sperm and increase the count and what do you think about artificial insemination and what are the chances in using my husband's sperm the way it is?

Comment—There are some things which can be done in certain instances to improve the sperm count (see answers to preceding letters).

As far as using the husband's sperm to induce artificial insemination, this is a possibility provided the proper facilities are available. Theoretically, if multiple sperm specimens were obtained, frozen, and saved, it would be possible to produce a large sperm specimen which could then be used for artificial insemination. Frozen sperm is only about two thirds as effective as live sperm so some potency would be lost on that account and if the original sperm cells were not motile or defective then they would probably not induce pregnancy anyway. But it is a possibility. When anatomical problems are the basis of the male sterility, such as an open urethral tube, then a collected specimen used for artificial insemination is sometimes successful.

116

VI

Masturbation

MASTURBATION MEANS INTENTIONAL SELF-STIMULATION for erotic pleasure, and it commonly occurs in animals as well as humans of both sexes. In the animal kingdom it has been observed in both sexes of rats, chinchillas, rabbits, porcupines, squirrels, parrots, horses, cows, elephants, dogs, baboons, monkeys, and chimpanzees.

In Kinsey's survey of women, about 60 percent acknowledged a history of masturbation, and approximately one-fifth of them were active within a year's span. It occurred usually about once a month among married females. Masturbation was the most important sexual outlet in single females, accounting for between 37 to 80 percent according to the age group. In married women it constituted about 10 percent of their sexual outlet. In older women who had previously been married, it was about 44 percent of their sexual outlet.

In an earlier study Dr. Catherine B. Davis obtained questionnaires from over 1,000 unmarried college graduates. Two thirds of these women reported a history of masturbation and one third of them had continued the practice. Of 1,000 married women, 40 percent reported masturbation. A breakdown of the age incidence of masturbation in the study showed that activity most commonly began between five and eleven years of age. Some began later. She reported 62 percent had experienced orgasm by masturbation around the age of eighteen. In commenting on female masturbation, Dr. Robert Dickinson, author of *Human Sex Anatomy,* stated, "Shall we then call auto-sexuality so general an experience or conduct as to be justly considered a normal provision of nature, as a stage preparatory for heterosexual response?"

Considering the incidence of masturbatory activity reported by the Kinsey survey in married women and in women who had previously been married, perhaps a better definition would be that it is a normal activity at interims throughout the female's life span.

It is now generally recognized that masturbation is normal in men. The Kinsey survey reported that it provided 71 percent of the sexual outlet in 85 percent of single men below fifteen years of age, and it remained the chief source of sexual outlet until marriage for men who later entered college. In single men in college it constituted about two-thirds of their sexual outlet. Their study also showed that among college graduate males about two-thirds of the married men occasionally masturbated, usually less than once or twice a week. At lower educational levels, married men masturbated less frequently. Thus masturbation in either the single or married male is not uncommon, and in fact, is the second most common form of sexual expression.

Despite the fact that most sex experts accept masturbation as common and a normal expression of sexuality, there still seems to be a great deal of ignorance about this subject. A study by Dr. Harold Lief concerning sexual education in medical schools demonstrated that half of the medical school seniors in one medical school in 1959 still thought that masturbation was the cause of insanity. Even worse, one-fifth of the faculty thought so too. This situation has significantly improved, and a more recent survey of the attitudes of physicians about sexual behavior indicated that about 90 percent of practicing physicians now accept masturbation as a normal means of sexual expression.

Masturbation, then, should be considered as normal activity. It does not cause pimples, insanity, knock-knees, homosexuality, or any number of ills that have been attributed to it. The greatest harm caused by masturbation is the psychic response or guilt feelings that many people have concerning the practice. This is a psychological response to the remnant of social disapproval. Some studies have suggested that women who masturbate are actually healthier than those who do not. One psychiatric text comments that if an individual reaches adult life without ever having experienced masturbation, the possibility of schizophrenia should be considered.

Masturbation is abnormal when it is carried out under inappropriate circumstances or in clearly excessive amounts. Then it becomes a symptom of an underlying problem rather than the cause of the difficulty. It is sometimes a symptom of anxiety. Sex acts as a soporific. Under anxiety-provoking situations, individuals may find relief from their anxiety through masturbation. An indication of the anxiety still caused by people's reaction to masturbation is evidenced by the many letters that I receive on this subject.

THE GIRLS

Dear Dr. Lamb—I am a fourteen-year-old girl with a question I hope you can answer. About two years ago I started to do something like masturbation. Does this occur among girls? It is a very good feeling. I fall asleep. Is it because it relaxes me? I get such satisfaction out of this that I am worried. Does this do anything to me? I have had my period only a few times, very irregularly and I wonder if it will be affected. What I do tickles and feels very good. Please explain and tell me what to do.

Comment—Many girls learn the technique of masturbation by self-examination and exploration. This girl apparently doesn't realize that this is a fairly common activity. There are numerous ways in which a girl can stimulate herself into an erotic state including stimulation of the breasts and the genitalia. The sensation of sleepiness after full sexual satisfaction is common. One of the things that achieving an or-

119

gasm accomplishes for a young woman is to relieve painful menstrual cramps. Masters and Johnson report that the orgasm is associated with a decrease in the pooling of blood and congestion in the female organs and relieves cramps observed in young women.

Dear Dr. Lamb—Is it unusual for a girl in her late teen-age years to have an uncontrollable desire for masturbation, even after injuring herself slightly and having to be taken to the hospital? How can this be overcome? Does she need a psychiatrist? Can this ruin her life? It's me and I'm worried and humiliated.

Comment—This is a typical reaction of an uninformed young girl. There seems to be a repeated cycle of feeling guilty, making efforts to control sexual activity, failure to be able to control such a strong drive, and then guilt for the act. None of this produces good mental health. It would be much better for a girl like this to understand that this is normal, but can be done to excess.

There are a number of ways a young girl can injure herself. Manipulation of the urethra is one way. All too often objects are poked into the urethra and this has not infrequently necessitated a trip to the hospital to retrieve pencils, cocktail stirrers, and other foreign objects.

Dear Dr. Lamb—Does masturbation change the appearance of the privates of a woman's body? Can a doctor tell by an examination whether or not a person has masturbated. What harm is caused by masturbation?

Comment—There is reason to believe that sexual activity in the woman can be strongly suspected at the time of physical examination. Dr. Robert Dickinson, author of *Human Sex Anatomy,* described a number of these observations which include changes in the size of the external genitalia, and with certain forms of activity, the size of the entrance to the vagina. The female who has not used tampons, a douche nozzle and has not experienced any form of sexual stimulation or insertion of any objects, finger or otherwise, has a

120

relatively small vagina that frequently will barely admit one finger at the time of initial insertion.

Far from being harmful to a woman, masturbation often prepares her for heterosexual life. The relaxation of the muscles that control the opening to the vagina and the stretching of the hymen will remove her fear of sexual activity and will enable her to approach her first heterosexual experiences with a decreased or minimal amount of difficulty. Many premarital examinations recommend exercises to women with a tight vagina and sensitive hymen to stretch the vaginal opening and hymen to prevent difficulties at the time of marriage. Also a study in women by Dr. Catherine Davis showed that a third of the women who continued masturbation were the healthiest, medically speaking. The only harm that masturbation can cause is when it is combined with some form of activity which can cause an injury, such as stimulating the urethral opening with a foreign object, or the use of other mechanical devices.

Dear Dr. Lamb—I am a seventeen-year-old girl. For as long as I can remember I have been practicing masturbation, so much that I have stretched my vaginal area. Would this keep me from reaching a climax later in married life? Is there any way that I can stop myself and is there anything that I can do about the shape of my vaginal area now?

Comment—The stretching of the vaginal area with certain forms of self-stimulation is natural. Nature has designed the female body in such a way that sexual stimulation will relax the muscles and prepare the area for heterosexual activity. Women who have enjoyed masturbation and have been able to reach a climax in this way are the ones who are most likely to enjoy heterosexual activity and reach a climax more easily. Some popular modern sex books have recommended that women who have difficulty in obtaining an orgasm should engage in self-stimulation under relaxing circumstances until they learn how to achieve one.

Although sexual organs that have been stimulated

121

frequently until they have undergone changes will regress to some extent and even the vaginal vault will decrease in size if it's not used, it will not return to the completely unstimulated tight opening and underdeveloped characteristics of the girl who has never had any form of sexual stimulation. To return to such a state, however, would be totally undesirable and unacceptable for heterosexual activity.

Dear Dr. Lamb—Is there any help for me? I have two boy cousins about three years older than I, and ever since I can remember they used me, but when I reached the age of eleven I rebelled. I quit, I said no more, I'm too big to do that. Now when I became a teen-ager I had a terrible sex urge but I never had relations with a male. I wanted to be a nice girl, so I would relieve myself. If only I had married when I was sixteen or seventeen, but no such luck. Do you think I can someday marry and have a normal life?

Comment—About all a girl with the normal sex urge that this girl describes needs to be married and enjoy a normal sex life is a willing husband.

OLDER WOMEN

Dear Dr. Lamb—I am a single woman aged sixty, who, a year ago, started masturbating out of a clear sky. Could drugs or medication bring on such a problem? The synthetic hormone, stilbestrol, which I took to control hot flashes for many years, was no longer effective and was discontinued. I was on mild doses of this hormone. Please advise me, as I am at a loss. There must be hormones to control the hot flashes other than the one I took.

Comment—It is quite common for women who have lost their sexual partner to find sexual relief by masturbation. The Kinsey studies bear this out as do many of the letters I receive. The only thing that can be wrong with this practice is one's moral attitude toward it. Since it relieves sexual tension, which in turn decreases excessive congestion of the female pelvic organs, it even has some beneficial effects to recommend it.

Dear Dr. Lamb—I am writing to you because of an item I saw in your column about a mother who was concerned about her son's masturbation. I have some middle-aged ladies rooming with me, and the case that concerns me is one who is seventy-six years of age. I find she is given to this habit quite frequently. What is the cause and is there a cure? She seems sensible and in all other ways normal, but I would like an explanation. Will this progress to any further trouble? If so, what is the remedy?

Comment—The best remedy is probably to let the lady have some privacy. Individuals do not lose their sexual urge throughout their life span and this woman is obviously living in circumstances that don't permit heterosexual expression of her sexual drive. It is not too surprising that she would engage in this form of activity. If all other aspects of her personality and living habits appear normal, there is no reason to regard such activity as indicative of any problem other than a strong sex drive that needs relief.

MOTHERS' QUESTIONS

Dear Dr. Lamb—I must say I am much relieved to have read your column that there is no harm in masturbation. You say a little is normal. My boy is eight and masturbates at least once a day, and some days twice that I know of. Is this excessive? Also I would like to know if twice a day is excessive for my daughter, aged ten, to masturbate.

Comment—Parents are often disturbed when they find that children are engaging in masturbation. This is true even though the parents themselves have at one time or another engaged in the same activity. Often their own masturbation was accompanied by guilt and this guilt is reawakened by their child's actions.

It is important that parents understand that masturbation is a normal expression of sexuality in children, and equally important that parents approach the subject properly with the child. This does not mean shaming them or criticizing them, but it does mean teaching them good manners in relationship to their sexual habits. This means that they should not be masturbating in public or engaging in any other unacceptable social behavior in public. This should be dealt with in the same manner that one teaches children other forms of good behavior, including good table manners, but it should not be construed as something that's going to be dangerous to the child. Specifically the child should not be told that masturbation will damage his sex life or cause him to be insane or any other such statements which will arouse severe anxiety. Statements of this sort are often very damaging to the child's psyche, because the child is going to continue to have strong sexual urges and will need to find some manner of sexual expression.

Dear Dr. Lamb—Can masturbation practiced through the teen years affect the process of growth? Some say yes, others say no. If not, does it have any other bad effects on the person besides that of guilt?

Comment—No, no, no, it does not affect growth. Masturbation does not cause physical harm to people unless it is associated with mechanical objects or use of devices that actually cause physical injury. Masturbation, both in animals and in man, is one form of normal sexual expression. It is not indicative of anything wrong with the individual, unless it is done under inappropriate circumstances and then it is a symptom and not a cause of difficulties.

Dear Dr. Lamb—Will you please tell me the dangers of masturbation. I am worried sick since I discovered our teen-age son doing it. We talked to him and told him

124

it was natural to experiment, but unhealthy to keep it up. Then I found out he was still doing it. I haven't told him I know. It's far too often, several nights a week. Can this lead to homosexuality?

Comment—About the only thing that the boy's masturbation will cause is a guilt complex, which will be reinforced by his mother's attitude. The worst thing that a parent can do is to implant the idea that masturbation leads to homosexuality. Since it's not likely that a young man with a strong sexual drive will lose this drive, the association of such ideas can be very harmful to the psyche. What's really needed here is education of the parents. Parents should also learn to respect the privacy of their children.

THE BOYS

Dear Dr. Lamb—I am in my middle teens and have gotten into a habit. I have been masturbating since twelve years of age. Sometimes I hold the sperm in by holding the main tube, but every so often I let it run out. My question is, could or would this have any effect on me or in having children later on in life?

Comment—Nothing could be further from the truth. Because of widespread ignorance many teen-agers are concerned that masturbation may affect their future sexual capacity. There also seems to be a widespread idea that the loss of seminal fluid will some way weaken the individual. The truth is that retention of the fluid in the male reproductive tract leads to engorgement and chronic inflammation of the prostate gland. The only harm that this young man can be doing himself is when he attempts to prevent the escape of seminal fluid at the time of orgasm. No doubt the pressure which is built up causes it merely to force the valve open at the outlet of the bladder and cause retrograde ejaculation of fluid into the bladder itself. He would be better off to let the fluid escape normally.

Dear Dr. Lamb—I am a male student, and I've been mas-

125

turbating four years now and have come to my senses and stopped this ridiculous act. Having indulged in it for so long, when I have tried to engage in intercourse (something you may not approve of at my age—I am in my teens), I've found that my penis will not get hard enough. My penis is bent from years of manipulation and will not and has not regained its former rigidity. If I can't find a way to enable it to become rigid, I think I might start masturbating again. My parents don't know about it and I'd rather they didn't. I haven't much money, but if a doctor or some pills would help I'd try to use them. The shape of my organ is really abnormal. I'd like your advice.

Comment—This boy's letter is a classic example of the bad effects of guilt about masturbation. This guilt complex can lead to problems with impotence. A little sensible counseling by a physician or a psychiatrist can usually relieve this problem.

The other factor which may be affecting this boy is simply inexperience in heterosexual activity. Time usually takes care of this difficulty.

While it's not clear what he means about the shape of his organ, and it's not likely he has very much information on the general shapes of erect organs to judge it properly, it is not true that masturbation significantly influences the shape of the organ. If masturbation increased the size of the penis, with the hangups that many men have on penis size, it would become a daily ritual. Many studies on the relationship of sexual activity and organ size have failed to show any relationship whatsoever between sexual activity and the size of the penis.

Dear Dr. Lamb—Last night I masturbated in the shower. I washed and wiped my hands, then washed my hair. My hands seemed free from sperm. In about two hours I had finger vaginal intercourse with my girl friend. I would like to know if there was any chance of my getting her pregnant from this. I am very worried.

126

Comment—This is an example of the extent of things which young people can worry about. It's most unlikely that after having washed the hands thoroughly, followed by washing the hair, that there would be any live sperm left on the hands. Thus it would seem unlikely that the young man's activity would induce pregnancy.

THE MEN

Dear Dr. Lamb—Would you please answer for me about masturbating. I do it for the purpose of discharging without getting involved with the opposite sex and getting VD. What damage am I causing myself? I remember doing this as far back as when I was fourteen years old, and I'm now forty-eight and the father of ten children. All are healthy, and I'm still going at it.

Comment—This man's record of ten children despite a life-long practice of sexual expression through masturbation should be ample evidence that masturbation does not cause sterility or impotence in the male. It is indeed one way of avoiding VD, as well as unwanted pregnancies.

Dear Dr. Lamb—I want your opinion. My next birthday I'll be seventy years of age. For obvious and financial reasons, and to satisfy my sex desires, I have been masturbating about one to three times a month for the last five years. I have no ill effects so far, and it seems to help me, for I do enjoy it. I have no trouble getting an erection. Please advise me if this will be harmful to me.

Comment—Many letters from readers in this age group indicate that masturbation is not uncommon in older men, thereby completing the entire age span and lending support to the concept that masturbation is a normal means of sexual expression.

Dear Dr. Lamb—I have masturbated off and on all my adult life. I am eighty-two years old, and I still mas-

127

turbate once a week. Is it true I could drop dead sometime after doing this? I suppose this is a silly question, but I'd like to know if I'd be healthier if I didn't do this. I feel very healthy as it is.

Comment—There is probably less likelihood for an older man to drop dead during masturbation than during sexual intercourse, particularly if he is having intercourse with someone besides his wife or regular sexual partner. Sexual activity of any sort increases the heart rate and blood pressure, but it has been demonstrated to increase the work of the heart more during extramarital affairs. There is no reason to suppose that masturbation is a significant health hazard in an individual who feels well enough to have a regular sustained sexual drive. There is some evidence that sexual activity increases the formation of testosterone, the male hormone, and to the extent that this maintains vitality in the male, continued sexual activity leading to orgasm may well be beneficial.

Dear Dr. Lamb—Why not be frank and tell us how many calories are used in masturbation? Calories are counted for everything these days including sexual intercourse, but for some strange reason, the calorie count for masturbation in men and women is ignored. Yet many say it affects our health and weight.

Comment—I doubt anyone really knows how many calories are used in masturbation. Techniques are quite varied, and require varied amounts of exertion and time. However, I can say that the probability of masturbation in a healthy person requiring so much exertion that it would cause any ill effects is quite remote and it's not likely to provide enough exercise to serve as an exercise for weight control.

IN MARRIAGE

Dear Dr. Lamb—As I am young I don't know of any other way to ask my question, and I'm too shy to ask someone what words I should use. I have been married a little less than one year. For some time now I have thought that my husband has been jacking off, but wasn't sure until today. I do know it isn't often, but it's too often for me. Does he do it because he doesn't have intercourse often enough or because when he does have intercourse he is not satisfied? I feel as though I have cheated him and feel cheated myself. I do hope you can answer, as I feel I might be the cause of his actions.

Comment—Judging from Kinsey and associates' studies on the incidence of masturbation in married men, this form of sexual behavior even in young men who've not been married too long is not unusual. It does, after all, provide a variety of sexual expression. It may well be one way that married men find a variety of sexual expression without becoming involved with another woman. In this way it actually helps to preserve the marriage.

Masturbation is more common in married men who have college educations, possibly because they are less apt to feel guilt or to believe the various myths associated with it. This activity in married men has little or nothing to do with the sexual satisfaction their wives provide, and the wife should not feel a sense of guilt if she realizes her husband occasionally enjoys this form of sexual expression. Likewise she should not feel that this is indicative of any less love for her or less sense of sexual attraction.

Under ideal circumstances between two intelligent, informed individuals, if both of them could come to understand the normality of a variety of sexual expression, a more healthy sexual outlook could be achieved. Basically, one of the reasons men do not continue to masturbate so frequently after marriage is that they find sexual intercourse more pleasurable.

Dear Dr. Lamb—I never thought I'd be asking you if you could answer a very personal question. Whatever makes a very nice man turn to masturbating? Luckily our youngsters are away for the summer or I would no

129

doubt have really fallen apart. He has been rather lax in the sex department for several months, but we talk freely to each other and he let me think he is just aging in his middle fifties. Some men do, but when I discovered why he has no pep it just about gave me a stroke. Is this a mental or physical thing that a doctor could help? I cannot talk to anyone about this and it's driving me mad. Please help me.

Comment—Obviously, masturbation should not be carried out to the exclusion of a satisfactory heterosexual relationship within a harmonious marriage. In some ways it represents a withdrawal of one of the partners from the other. Nevertheless the simple act of a married man masturbating does not mean that he is abnormal as is indicated by the figures on the incidence of masturbation conducted by Kinsey. If both partners realize that such activity is normal and are able to discuss it freely, the probabilities of such activity causing a serious breakup in a marriage will be minimized.

Dear Dr. Lamb—My problem, I fully realize, is by no means unique, but the fact remains it has really affected my mental state and my marriage. Several years ago I married for a second time a man with whom I thought I could be happy. Now I truly love my husband and want to save my marriage. My husband says he loves me too and I believe this is so. The problem is my husband masturbates frequently. I made the mistake of deciding to talk it over with my husband, and he blew his stack. We ended up shouting and screaming at each other and him threatening a divorce.

In the past he has been good sexually. He was a bit like a jackrabbit at first, but after a time he settled down to a satisfactory sexual relationship. But with this new habit I'm left with the short end of the stick, so to speak. Intercourse is only at the most once a week, and sometimes every two weeks.

I had the same problem with my first husband. However, I thought it was more important that I was

130

a virgin bride and thought that his masturbation was the real solution. But when it continued after marriage and even on our wedding night, I was very disillusioned. It caused a lot of problems, and finally we were separated and I don't wish to make the same mistake again. I have resolved to do whatever is necessary to better please my husband and show him how much I love him, and hope that in the long run he will realize this and our problem will work itself out. Sometimes it is very difficult for me to do. Could you give me some urgently needed advice?

Comment—This type of problem can certainly be frustrating for a woman who enjoys and needs more sexual activity. Although surveys suggest that masturbation within marriage is quite normal, no sexual activity should be allowed to interfere with the mutual sexual satisfaction of both parties within the marriage. No doubt problems of this nature deserve discussion with a competent marriage counselor or a psychiatrist.

In situations like this, though, it is often difficult to talk the other partner into seeking counsel. The best advice I can give for women with this problem is to go see a psychiatrist. They'll need support anyway while they are living through such a frustrating experience. While seeing a psychiatrist, a woman may be able to obtain some help in getting her mate into a counseling situation. It is far better for the wife to do this than to nag or confront the husband.

Begging, pleading, nagging, and accusing all seem to make these situations worse and cause the wife to be less desirable or sexually attractive to the man, which merely aggravates the situation rather than resolving the problem. This requires restraint on the part of the wife and she will be well advised to merely tell her husband that she is very distressed and nervous and wants to see a psychiatrist. After she has obtained her initial interviews with the psychiatrist and entered into consultation, she can depend upon the advice of her psychiatrist as to the best course of action to follow thereafter.

I receive a number of letters from women who are deeply concerned about their husbands' masturbation. Incidentally, I do not receive any letters from men who are concerned about their wives' masturbation. Since studies show that married women do masturbate, this strongly suggests that they are more successful in preventing their husband from knowing it (after all, they are at home all day) or else their husbands are less concerned.

Dear Dr. Lamb—What would make a man in his early forties turn from his wife for seemingly no reason and use himself for sex fulfillment. I lie awake night after night while he enjoys himself. I do not imagine this, as it has been going on now for several months. At first only once in a while, but now it is almost every night. I feel his movements and hear the sound, even see the movement of his body until I think I will fly apart from wanting him so badly. I know of no reason. I try to look nice for him and do what is expected, plus a lot that I know is not expected of me. I have tried to talk to him, only to be treated like I am unclean.

I enjoy sex and love him very much, but at night that love turns to hate when he does this thing. My nerves are about shot, but he doesn't seem to notice or maybe he doesn't care. We have children which he loves very much, and at times I feel he still loves me, but he has said things I would not have believed he would ever say to me, like he wants to hurt me. But I don't know why. I try to ignore what happens at night, but I just can't. I hate to see darkness come. I'm lucky if he wants me once in two weeks' time. If he does have sex relations with me, he doesn't really want to, but acts as though he's duty-bound.

Sometimes he lies so close to me when he satisfies himself that I feel every movement. Other times he places a pillow between us. I tried once to ignore what was going on and make love to him. He drew away and was very angry and talked terrible to me, as

132

though I had no right to be there.

I must add in the daytime he is very good to me, and I want for nothing, but I think his complete indifference the night before is hurting me as much as anything. He acts as though nothing had happened and expects me to act the same way. God knows I do try, but it's the hardest thing I have ever had to face in my life. I've read everything I can find about this problem, but nothing is presented in detail. Can you help me to learn if this may be a phase of manhood of which I know little or can it go on indefinitely? I certainly cannot.

Comment—I would suggest that this couple should see a psychiatrist for support during this emotionally trying period in their lives. It is often wise within the marriage, if one of the partners is having serious emotional difficulties and will not seek help, for the other partner to seek some help themselves. This, at least, makes the situation easier to bear and sometimes leads to bringing both partners into professional counseling with good results for all concerned.

VII

Homosexuality, Male and Female

ALTHOUGH IT IS DIFFICULT for individuals conditioned to the Judeo-Christian culture to realize it, homosexual acts are an accepted form of sexual expression in many other cultures. In commenting on the uniquely severe attitudes in our culture about homosexuality, Kinsey and collaborators made this historical observation:

> The more general condemnation of all homosexual relationships originated in Jewish history in about the seventh century B.C., upon the return from the Babylonian exile. Both mouth-genital contacts and homosexual activities had previously been associated with the Jewish religious service, as they had been with the religious services of most of the other peoples of that part of Asia, and just as they have been in many other cultures elsewhere in the world. . . . Jewish sex codes were brought over into Christian codes by the early adherents of the Church, including St. Paul, who had been raised in the Jewish tradition on matters of sex.

Within our culture at least three clearly identified schools of thought exist concerning homosexuality. One group, the behavioral scientists, looked for the explanation by trying to see how animals, primitive man, various cultures and modern man actually behave. From these observations they de-

134

duce what seem to be the natural forms of sexual expression. The Kinsey approach belongs to this group.

A second group uses the psychoanalytic approach, which gained much of its original impetus from the early work of Freud. This has always been more of a theoretical approach commonly based on intensive studies of individual cases. Because Freudian theories are not supported by the amount of factual observations used by the behavioral group nor the exactness of a pure science such as biochemistry, they have always been suspected of being more fanciful than factual. Its philosophic roots are deep in Judeo-Christian ethics with all of their cultural implications. This is one reason why much Freudian philosophy has not been applicable to other cultures such as those of Asia, Africa, and the Middle East. The concept of sexual guilt in many of these cultures is without meaning.

The third group approach sexuality on a genetic-chemical basis. They find correlations between the ratio of male and female hormones or hormonal influences during fetal development and even chromosomal variations as explanations for sexual behavior.

It is not likely that something as complex as sexual behavior will be properly explained by one simple concept. No doubt basic behavioral patterns, psychiatric factors, and genetic-chemical factors are all applicable in varying degrees of importance in any one individual.

The comments of Kinsey and his collaborators are of particular importance in view of the large amount of extensive data they accumulated in both men and women. In attempting to cover the entire behavioral field, this group pointed up other studies concerning the sexual behavior in animals. In this regard, they stated:

> In actuality, sexual contacts between individuals of the same sex are known to occur in practically every species of mammal which has been extensively studied. In many species, homosexual contacts may occur with considerable frequency, although never as frequently as heterosexual contacts.

These observations applied to both male and female animals.

In looking at the frequency of homosexuality in females, the Kinsey group estimated that homosexual activity occurred in 28 percent of American women. Homosexual acts occurred most frequently in unmarried women or women who had been previously married. Nevertheless, homosexual tendencies were found to be present in 8 to 10 percent of married women. These figures were somewhat lower than the corresponding figures for men. However, this finding is subject to interpretation of what constitutes a homosexual act. In the American culture many acts between women are socially acceptable, such as hugging and kissing, while these same acts between men would be considered as homosexual activity. This is not necessarily true of many other cultures.

The Kinsey studies provided information which led the authors to state that homosexual activity to the point of orgasm occurred in approximately 37 percent of American men between adolescence and old age. Their study showed that it was much more common in unmarried men or previously married men than in those who were married. However, the histories of unmarried men indicated frequent activity or contacts with a larger segment of married men than was indicated from the interviews with married men themselves. This discrepancy casts some doubt on the accuracy of the figures for married men. It should also be added that since the Kinsey studies were based on face-to-face interviews there is good reason to suspect that the incidence of these forms of sexual activity are actually much higher in the American population than is indicated by the studies. The remarkable thing about the Kinsey survey is the relatively high incidence of a wide variety of sexual behavior that was acknowledged in a face-to-face interview, particularly since many of these forms of activity are punishable offenses by currently existing legal statutes.

In interpreting their data in men and women, the comments of the Kinsey group are important. The highlights are therefore included.

In view of the data which we now have on the in-

136

cidence and frequency of the homosexual, and in particular on his coexistence with the heterosexual in the
lives of a considerable portion of the male population, it is difficult to maintain the view that psycho-
sexual reactions between individuals of the same sex
are rare and therefore abnormal or unnatural, or
that they constitute within themselves evidence of
neuroses or even psychoses.

The investigators go on to emphasize that the existence of
these forms of activity on such a scale in view of the general
attitude of the public regarding these activities was a strong
indication of the fundamental drive in this area.

They further observed:

. . . its wide occurrence today in some cultures in
which such activity is not as taboo as it is in our own,
suggests that the capacity of an individual to respond
erotically to any sort of stimulus, whether it is provided by another person of the same or the opposite
sex, is basic in the species.

The mammalian record thus confirms our statement that any animal which is not too strongly conditioned by some special sort of experience is capable
of responding to any adequate stimulus. This is what
we find in the more uninhibited segments of our own
human species, and this is what we find among
young children who are not too rigorously restrained
in their early sex play. Exclusive preferences and patterns of behavior, heterosexual or homosexual, come
only with experience, or as a result of social pressures which tend to force an individual into an exclusive pattern of one or the other sort.

And, finally, the authors comment:

. . . considering the physiology of sexual response
and mammalian backgrounds of human behavior, it
is not so difficult to explain why a human animal
does a particular thing sexually. It is more difficult
to explain why each and every individual is not involved in every type of sexual activity.

Certainly, homosexuality has been around a long time. The ancient culture of Sparta is commonly cited as an example of a homosexual culture. Stanley Pacion, a historian, commenting on Plutarch's Sparta, observed that while it might not be entirely factual it was not fiction either, and pointed out that the translation to English had been curiously sanitized to de-emphasize the obvious fact that the nation of Sparta regulated the sexual lives of its citizens. In fact, the culture was based on homosexuality with de-emphasis on heterosexuality. In analyzing the reason for this, homosexuality was used as a means of preserving the state. The male lovers bore a responsibility for each other's acts, good or bad, which helped to strengthen the camaraderie and feeling necessary for the invincible fighting forces of Greece. Every twelve-year-old boy of promise in Sparta already had a lover to bear him company. Marriages were encouraged, but the bride's hair was shorn and the man saw her in the bridal chamber after dark, fulfilled his sexual obligation, and returned to the barracks. The children belonged to the state. Such patterns of sexual behavior clearly emphasize the role of cultural influences in shaping behavior. It is not likely that this form of behavior would occur naturally without extraneous influences.

It is not necessary to turn to ancient Greece to find examples of socially approved homosexuality. In our own Southwest homosexual activity was openly approved among the female Mojave Indians. In all of these cultures, however, which are labeled as homosexual, male or female, it is obvious that there was a major bisexual element; otherwise, the culture could not have continued.

There are numerous examples in history of prominent individuals who engaged in a variety of sexual activity. Although Julius Caesar was notorious for his sexual prowess and rumor had him sleeping with the wife of every important political person in Rome, his earlier days were clouded by a history of homosexual activity. Stanley Pacion, in commenting on this, referred to Cicero's writing, "Caesar was led by Nicomedes' attendants to the royal bedchamber, where he lay on a golden couch, dressed in purple shift—so this descendent of Venus lost his virginity in Bithynia." Nicodemes' Oriental court was known for its free-wheeling, uninhibited sexual activity.

Plutarch, in writing of the life of Julius Caesar, also makes note almost inferentially of the homosexual activity among Roman women. He recounts an episode involving Caesar's wife, Pompeia. The occasion was a religious ceremony when all of the men were to be out of the living quarters where the women were enacting the religious rites. The beardless Roman Claudius dressed like a woman and stole into the quarters to have a rendezvous with Pompeia. Plutarch recounts that while Claudius was in the quarters waiting for Pompeia, he was approached by one of the maids, who "invited him to play with her, as the women did among themselves. He refused to comply, and she presently pulled him forward, and asked him who he was and whence he came." Claudius betrayed himself by his voice. The important observation here is the accepted freedom of the women's activities with each other, which led to the unmasking of Claudius, the man impersonating a woman.

Bisexual behavior is common today and, as Dr. David E. Smith of the Haight-Asbury free medical clinic observed, it is commonly encountered in some hippie cultures and is described as being "AC/DC." Dr. Smith repeats the philosophy to be "as one young person said, you should be able to love everybody, whether he is a man or a woman. Sex is the greatest, and if everybody would have sexual relations then there would be a lot less hate." By this definition, hate and hostility result from suppression of the natural sex drive.

There are numerous examples of homosexual activity in both men and women during confinement. In one study of fifty-seven delinquent, adolescent girls, 69 percent reported being involved in "girl stuff." A comparable study in male adolescents indicated that over 50 percent had some form of homo-erotic activity while imprisoned. Some of these forms of activity are clearly symbiotic means of relief of sexual tensions with the only possible partner available under confinement. More recently, Jimmy Hoffa has also commented on the frequency of the first night homosexual rape of newly admitted inmates.

Perhaps one of the most prominent women to have been known for her bisexual activity was George Sand. She took a masculine name and wore men's clothing. She made no secret of her love for Marie Dorval, and her letters were full of her passion. However, she was equally at home in a heterosexual role and lived happily with a series of male geniuses, including Chopin.

Clearly there is abundant evidence of a human tendency to engage in a variety of sexual expressions which is neither exclusively heterosexual nor homosexual, and is markedly influenced by the norms a particular culture has established. These observations all lend heavy support to the concept of the behavioral scientists concerning the capacity of the human species to respond to sexual stimulation of any type, regardless of its source, given the appropriate circumstances.

Even though behavioral studies of animals and people in a variety of cultures show homosexual behavior to be common, one must not lose sight of the obvious, that heterosexual expression is the most frequent form of sexual activity.

As a rule, psychiatrists tend to believe that homosexual tendencies are encouraged by a dominant mother who often develops a special relationship with her son, whereas the father is absent, weak, withdrawn, or in some instances sufficiently hostile as to be forbidding. A similar but opposite pattern sometimes is advanced for homosexuality in the female. Dr. Henry Biller of the University of Rhode Island points out, "girls who feel devalued and rejected by their fathers are more likely to become homosexuals than are girls whose fathers are warm and accepting."

Despite these stereotyped patterns of family background used to explain sexual behavior, a number of studies have shown that these classic parental situations do not always apply. Similar patterns can be found in individuals who are not thought to engage in any form of homosexual activity (in both men and women) and likewise, the classic parental pat-

140

terns are frequently absent in individuals who are known to engage regularly in homosexual activity. Much remains to be learned about the psychiatric influences that early family life exerts on the individual. There is sufficient evidence, however, to realize that it is an important factor in shaping the outcome of sexual identity, even though it may not be the exclusive factor.

Not all psychiatrists follow the classic dogma. Dr. Martin Hoffman, psychiatrist in San Francisco, states that, contrary to the opinion held by many psychiatrists, he does not regard homosexual activity as an illness. "I regard homosexuals as members of an oppressed minority group rather than as mentally ill." He rejects the idea that individuals who engage in homosexual acts can be cured by psychotherapy, and compares this measure to the question of "What outcome can be expected in psychotherapy of Jews?" It is safe to say that the large and growing body of factual information on the gamut of sexual behavior has had and is continuing to have a forceful impact on previously held psychiatric viewpoints.

While chemical studies of the relationship of male and female hormones have failed to provide any differentiation between individuals who engage in both heterosexual and homosexual activity, there have been a number of studies that have indicated that individuals who engage exclusively in homosexual activity tend to have an abnormal endocrine pattern. A study currently in process by Masters and Johnson from apparently well-adjusted males in this category suggest that they may have a decrease in testosterone, or male hormone, levels. Those individuals who engage in all forms of sexual activity, or exclusively heterosexual activity, may have more normal hormone chemistries. Similar studies involving the same general problems, but different types of measurements, have been reported by other investigators. Dr. Sidney Margolese, of Los Angeles, in collaboration with psychiatrists and psychologists, was one of the earlier scientists to demonstrate the probability that hormonal levels could indeed be important at least in some individuals who engaged exclusively in homosexual acts. Disturbances in hormone functions during pregnancy have been identified as a factor in gender behavior in animals. Scientists think the hormone disturbances affect the early development of the brain and hence gender identification.

It is no wonder with this degree of confusion about what's normal and what's not normal, what's moral and what's immoral, what's sick and what's healthy, that the general public might be somewhat confused about homosexual activity. I would like to make one generalization that furthering of understanding might be accomplished by eliminating labels. Because an individual engages in a homosexual act does not mean that he is a homosexual any more than a person who engages in a heterosexual act is a heterosexual. A person is a person, an act is an act.

Unfortunately, many individuals who have been labeled as homosexuals have, by virtue of the labeling, been forced into a form of life-style somewhat different from that which they might otherwise have enjoyed within society. If a young boy should be caught in a homosexual act, the very knowledge that he has done this is apt to sharply limit his heterosexual opportunities in the future, thereby defining his future life-style.

Telling a person that he or she is a homosexual has somewhat the same impact as telling a child that he has no ability in mathematics. The child will begin to believe he has no capacity in mathematics and, therefore, he won't have. If a girl is told she is a homosexual and cannot enjoy a heterosexual life, she will believe that this is true, and the same applies to a boy. Therefore, one should exercise particular care to use the phrase "homosexual acts" or "homosexual activity," and not confuse this with the label of the individual, as if he belonged to a special ethnic group. I receive a limited number of letters on homosexual problems simply because many people are afraid of the problem. Others are satisfied with their solution, and many others really don't expect any help. Nevertheless the letters that do arrive clearly exemplify the concern over this problem that exists in our society.

142

THE MOTHER

Dear Dr. Lamb—I am a frantic mother who needs some help on homosexuals. I have just found out that my twenty-five-year-old son is a homosexual. Please give me any information that you can on this. Is there any help for them? Will psychiatric help be of any assistance? Is there any kind of help they can get? What are some of their characteristics? Is there such a thing as just having homosexual inclinations mildly? Are they born, or is it something that develops while they are growing up? Can they be successful in the business world, or does this thing become a great worry and sorrow to them? Can they live a normal life as a bachelor and ignore sex? Please answer me.

Comment—Imagine the real frustration and anxiety this mother must feel. Remember that there is probably no one in her immediate social circle whom she can discuss this vital problem with. What she really means about her son being a homosexual would require probing. If, indeed, he is having any type of problem or anxiety about his sexual activity, he should see a competent psychiatrist. Even though many psychiatrists are still struggling with their own understanding of how to deal with the spectrum of sexual activity, it is still the best opportunity currently available to him.

Many young people who imagine they are "homosexuals" are merely experiencing normal feelings. Dr. Paul Fink of Hahnemann Medical College, commented on one aspect of this in describing the case of an eighteen-year-old male who was very disturbed by certain erotic feelings toward a male friend. In Dr. Fink's opinion, this is relatively normal, particularly in early years. He comments, "The revival of early feelings of an erotic nature, which in infancy occur regardless of the actual gender of the object, is frightening when they occur toward people of the same sex." Dr. Fink points out that this can prevent friendships because of the fear that individuals of the same sex have when they find that they are responding to someone of their own gender, even though the feelings themselves are never acted upon.

143

The lady's question about the characteristics of the "homosexual" is typical. Many individuals who engage in homosexual acts, both men and women, present no characteristics that distinguish them from their associates, appearing in all aspects to be ordinary men and women. While it is common to think of the man who engages in homosexual activity as being effeminate and the woman as being a "butch," these standard characterizations have little relationship to reality. In fact, many effeminate men and many "butch" women lead exclusively heterosexual lives. Of course, there are all levels of homosexual activity.

Dear Dr. Lamb—Would you tell me about homosexuality? My generation knew nothing about such, but now my family is being affected by this problem. Can a homosexual father a child? Do they get over it? Can they be treated by a doctor? Does it affect them mentally? What should be the attitude of society toward them? Please tell me everything you can. I have no one to turn to. One of my close relatives married a lovely girl, and it lasted about a week. Another relative's husband turned out to be a homosexual. One of the teachers in the school system also had it, and I suspect there are more boys involved in this than we know.

Comment—This lady's letter exemplifies many of the misconceptions about individuals who engage in homosexual activities. Using Kinsey's statistics, it is clear that a large percentage of men who have at one time or another engaged in homosexual acts are fathers. The ability to have children and one's sexual behavior are not necessarily related. Nor does one's sexual activity affect one mentally. Quite the contrary, most psychiatrists feel that unusual sexual behavior is often a symptom of a psychiatric problem rather than a cause.

As to whether individuals who commit homosexual acts get over this form of behavior or not, one could obtain a variety of opinions. I am sure that those individuals who consider homosexual behavior merely one aspect of normal sexual expression would regard this somewhat in the same light

144

as getting over being Jewish, Italian, or Anglo-Saxon. Psychiatrists who consider homosexual behavior as an illness, however, report that a number of individuals' behavior has been altered, although most acknowledge that this is a difficult goal to achieve.

It is important to point out that psychiatric treatment for this purpose does not change the person's personality or character so much, but rather changes the sexual behavior. Such a change in sexual behavior may be very advantageous in most segments of the Judeo-Christian culture, but would not necessarily be important in other cultures.

There is no unanimity of opinion regarding society's attitude toward homosexual activity for either men or women. No doubt if society accepted homosexual acts as merely one other form of sexual expression, it would not greatly affect the overall sexual orientation of the majority of people. Clear evidence for this point is established in societies where it is not condemned, and yet in all of these, despite intermittent episodes of homosexual acts, heterosexual activity remains the dominant form of expression. Even when homosexual acts are not condemned, most mature adults in those societies adopt heterosexual activity as their principal means of sexual expression, although it may not be their exclusive or only means of sexual expression. Heterosexuality is chosen without excluding warm relationships between individuals of the same sex, or even on occasion, sexual expression. Thus if our society condoned homosexual acts, it would not likely decrease significantly the present frequency of heterosexual activity.

THE BOY

Dear Dr. Lamb—I am twenty-one years old. I am a homosexual. I want help so I can have a wife and children. I have heard of a doctor who operates on homosexuals to make them well. Do you know of this doctor, and do you know if there is such an operation? What would happen if I went to my doctor? What would he do with me? Is there any hope for me?

Comment—There have been and are studies going on utilizing even brain surgery in an attempt to convert individuals' sexual behavior to a heterosexual pattern. Success has been reported by some investigators in this area. It is true that the brain can significantly affect the type of sexual behavior in an individual, but whether or not this means that a surgical approach would be appropriate in an individual who engages in homosexual acts is not established. Even so, there are probably a number of individuals in whom it would not be appropriate. Using the Kinsey statistics it would seem unlikely that nearly 40 percent of the American male population should be subjected to brain surgery. This is approximately the frequency of individuals who have, at one time or another, engaged in one or more homosexual acts between adolescence and old age.

Doctors often react as individuals when they are confronted with a patient who admits to performing homosexual acts. Usually these reactions are a mirror of society, since doctors are members of society and subject to the same kind of responses. Frankly, most doctors do not view homosexual acts objectively. Even those who intellectually believe that it is either an illness or normal behavioral pattern still react emotionally and adversely when confronted. Not all doctors are enlightened on sexual behavior. Most family doctors, however, do recognize that homosexual play in both girls and boys in their developmental stage is a normal aspect of childhood and are not so likely to panic if the mother brings in a young child, greatly disturbed about what she has seen during play activities.

THE GIRL

Dear Dr. Lamb—I'm not sure how to write this letter to you or even if I should, but I need help and I couldn't possibly talk to my doctor about it, so I'm hoping you can help me. The problem is with my girl friend. We've been good friends since we were in high school

146

and now we are both twenty-four and we've been very close friends all these years.

Well, she got married about a year ago to this guy who seemed like a real nice man. Then they started having trouble. My friend didn't enjoy having sex with him, but that didn't stop him. He wanted to have sex almost every night. Things went from bad to worse and she left him. She didn't have any place to go, so when they separated she moved in with me which was fine since we could share the rent.

The apartment is small and it only has one bedroom with a double bed. You have probably already guessed what I'm going to tell you. She was very emotional and upset about her broken marriage. She claimed the reason she didn't want sex with her husband was because he drank before going to bed, and she just couldn't stand the smell of alcohol on him when he started to make love to her.

Because she was so emotional, I tried to comfort her and be affectionate. She seemed to want more and more. At night she would hug me and kiss me before we went to sleep. Well, one thing led to another and pretty soon she was massaging my breasts and stimulating me sexually. Now she has become sexually aggressive with me and wants me to do the same with her. She says it is perfectly all right because she loves me. I don't know whether she is sick or whether I am. I don't want to hurt her, but I don't want to live a bad life either. What can I do?

Comment—When individuals go through emotional crises in their lives, they often reach out for emotional support from other people. The need to be loved seems to be universal to the human species, and with that comes a need to express the love or be reassured of love. Sex is a powerful means of communicating. The situation described by this girl is not unique. The factors related to an unsuccessful marriage and unsuccessful adjustment to heterosexual activity indicate a need for professional help. The biggest tragedy evidenced by

147

this letter is not so much the homosexual activity between the two girls, but the failure to be able to enjoy normal heterosexual activity, and the opportunity for normal family life and the rearing of children.

THE WIFE

Dear Dr. Lamb—I have been married for twenty years to a homosexual (this he will not admit; however, he has been caught before). For fifteen years we had sexual activity occasionally and we have several children who are all grown now. For the past five years my husband has been impotent, as far as I am concerned. He has become depressed, sick, and even mean at times to me. His attitude is almost unbearable. Would this be because he is not able to have his contacts with homosexuals now, or is it still possible that he is having homosexual activity, but am I to blame? What I would really like to know is, is it possible for a man to have homosexual relations and still not be able to have relations with his wife?

Comment—Certainly, just as a man can have successful sex relations with another woman and be impotent with his wife, it's entirely possible for him to have sexual activity with another man and be impotent with his wife. The problem of impotence is complex and will be discussed in a separate chapter. I would add, however, that it's common for a man who suffers impotency to be depressed and sick and under these circumstances, I suppose "even mean."

It's worth observing that many women, when their husbands do not satisfy them sexually or otherwise appear not to be giving them the attention they think they deserve, accuse their husbands of homosexuality, whether this is true or not. This has a double-barreled effect of making the man guilty and therefore responsible for the difficulties in the marriage, while at the same time exonerating the wife from any contribution she may have made to the marital difficulties.

148

Individuals who have a serious conflict about their own homosexual drives are more apt to accuse others of such behavior or to have an aggressively negative attitude toward homosexual acts. Such a wife may have had a strong attachment for a female childhood friend or have experienced homosexual acts in her own past. Men also, who are excessively hostile about others' homosexual acts, often have the same conflict, consciously or unconsciously.

Since homosexual acts are viewed with such great alarm in American society, this is a very useful and effective weapon for a wife to use against her husband, particularly if he is not very secure in his own masculinity and feels threatened by such accusations. Men are less likely to accuse their wives of homosexual activity because many of the forms of expressing affection between two women are socially accepted.

Dear Dr. Lamb—I think I am married to a homosexual. I am a loving wife and have tried since we were married to have my husband make love to me. In the several years we have been married he doesn't even put his arms around me or caress me in any way. Even on our honeymoon we slept in twin beds. I thought at first this was just because he was shy. This didn't bother me because I am a shy person myself. Before we got married when he kissed me he used to put his tongue in my mouth and this seemed to give him a thrill. I didn't like it and told him so. We didn't have intercourse until after the honeymoon. After a few times, he wasn't interested in me any more. I've tried to discuss this with him but he won't talk to me and so we live like two strangers underneath the same roof, polite but we have no companionship. Does any of this sound like what I am suspicious of? How can one tell? I would never let him know that I knew if this is true.

Comment—This woman is jumping to conclusions. There could be a number of reasons why a healthy sex life has not developed after marriage. The real problem cannot be identified and dealt with without professional counseling. If she rebuffed the man's sexual advances because she didn't like his manner of kissing or by other ways indicated a lack of interest in sexual activity, she may indeed have affected the early development of their sexual life. The man may have some other problem, including impotency. It is usually a poor idea for a wife to speculate that her husband's problem with sexual activity has a homosexual basis. There are plenty of other reasons why a man could have trouble adjusting sexually. The identification of a problem shouldn't be done by a wife without medical or psychiatric training, but rather by a competent professional.

THE FRIEND

Dear Dr. Lamb—I am a very worried mother. My son is fifteen. I am not concerned about his dating girls, but it's this feeling he has about a twenty-two-year-old boy. My son wants to be with this older boy every chance he gets. He even thinks up things to tell him when he's with him. I do not know what they do when alone and I cannot guess, but I do want to know if it is normal to be so taken with one of your own sex. If not, what do I do with my son?

Comment—This letter points out how uptight American society is about homosexual acts. According to this mother's letter, she has no real evidence or reason to think that anything more than a deep friendship exists between her son and an older boy. It's not uncommon for young boys to have an older hero—movie stars, football stars, baseball players, sometimes more tangible ones, but they are heroes.

Unless one has good reason to feel that an offspring is maladjusted or having emotional difficulties, parents are well advised not to interfere with the friendships their children develop as long as their associates are respectable individuals with respectable habits.

Parents who are overly concerned about every friendship that their children develop often have reasons within their own emotional makeup to experience undue anxiety, and often it is their problem and not the child's. The same is true of many individuals who assume or concern themselves about the sexual activity of others. Sometimes these exaggerated, unhealthy interests are a symptom of the raging sexual conflict, conscious or unconscious, in the mind of the gossiper or the accuser.

Perhaps the best protection against having an offspring slip into homosexual activity as an exclusive means of sexual expression is to be certain that he is adequately surrounded by members of the opposite sex. Many psychiatrists believe that a key element in the individual's personality who engages exclusively in homosexual activity is a phobic reaction to members of the opposite sex. As with most things in life, the unknown is feared and the known is understood, tolerated or enjoyed. Since men and women are destined to spend their lives together under one social arrangement or another, the sooner the sexes get to know each other the better they will be able to either cope with each other or enjoy each other as the case may be.

VIII

Impotence
and Related Problems

SEXUAL FAILURE, for whatever reason, is greatly distressing to either the male or the female. It strikes at the ego, making a person feel inferior and less of a man or a woman. Sexual failure in the male is known as impotence. It means failure to maintain an erect penis long enough to satisfactorily complete sexual intercourse. Related conditions which are sometimes included with impotence are premature ejaculation, where the man reaches an orgasm before he is able to satisfactorily provide stimulation for his sexual partner, and the rare condition of orgasmic failure, where the man may maintain an erection but fail to have an orgasm.

ERECTION FAILURE

There is no way that a man can hide the condition of his flaccid organ when he wants to have sexual relations and the penis does not respond. A woman, however, can hide her dysfunction by relaxing and taking a passive role. The penis is a singularly independent organ. Not only does it fail to respond at the urging of its owner, but on other occasions it responds too vigorously, much to the owner's embarrassment. During the time of Leonardo da Vinci, this gave rise to the idea that the penis had a separate brain or mind of its own. Leonardo da Vinci's comments on the independent nature of the penis gave rise to speculation that he himself may have suffered from impotence. Having read these translations, however, I must say that it is equally plausible that he was complaining about the independent, persistent erection which most men have experienced from one time to another with varying degrees of social embarrassment.

Impotence is a fairly common complaint. Immediately after orgasm, the male is usually impotent for a short period of time. No stranger to any man, this form of impotence is a normal body response unrelated to psychological factors or disease of any type. Relatively persistent impotence that interferes with a man's capacity for sexual intercourse is less common, although many physicians think the problem is sharply increasing in American men.

It is estimated that at least 2 percent of young men thirty-five years of age or younger are impotent, and that by the age of fifty-five impotence affects 10 percent. At seventy-five years of age and beyond, 50 percent of men are impotent, which incidentally also means that 50 percent retain their sexual powers. These figures are only estimates because the true incidence of impotency is not known. It is not something that men discuss readily.

The apparent increase of impotence in young, otherwise healthy American men has been attributed by Dr. George L. Ginsberg, a New York psychiatrist, and his colleagues to the Women's Liberation movement and the general sexual liberation of women who, rather than being passive partners, now demand standards of performance from their men. In the Victorian era a man's impotence could merely be attributed to an unwillingness to impose on his sexually disinterested wife.

While it is difficult to obtain accurate figures on the longevity of potency, it is interesting to note that many men remain potent until they are advanced in years. There are sufficient records of individuals who have fathered children in their nineties to substantiate this point, and autopsy examinations have found live sperm cells in the prostates of men considered elderly by current standards.

In societies relatively free of heart disease, strokes, and

other manifestations of fatty deposits in the arteries (atherosclerosis), it is common for older men to retain their sexual capacity. It is not unusual for a male Abkhasian to remain sexually active until the age of one hundred. One case reported that a man one hundred and nineteen years of age was fully potent, and a semen examination demonstrated quantities of live sperm adequate to father a child.

One of the ignored contributing factors to impotency in the American society is the incidence of atherosclerosis, or fatty deposits in the arteries, the same disease that causes heart disease and strokes. The Armed Forces Institute of Pathology reports that the testicles are one of the earliest organs to be affected by atherosclerosis. In older patients this reverses the male-female hormone levels. Put simply, our living habits (overeating, excessive fat in the diet, particularly saturated fats or animal fats, high cholesterol intake, lack of exercise, cigarette smoking, excessive use of alcohol and coffee), through contributing to the early development of atherosclerosis in the American male, can be an important factor in loss of sexual capacity relatively early in life.

The blood supply to the testicles is unique. The arteries spread out over the surface of the testicles; then the branches of the arteries turn very sharply in a right, or acute, angle to enter the body of the testicle. Sharp angulations of this type in the arteries are particularly prone to develop fatty deposits. No doubt there are psychological reasons for impotence in the younger American males and no doubt with the greater understanding of these problems, many of these men are seeking help who previously didn't bother to do so, but one should not lose sight of the probability that poor circulation to the testicles may be a real factor in the apparent decrease in potency in American males. The fatty deposits in the arteries, by affecting the parts of the testicles that are responsible for the formation of sperm, also may contribute to low sperm counts or male sterility.

It is recognized that decreased amounts of male hormones can decrease a man's sex drive. This may be enough to tip the balance in a marginal situation. A little more male hormone, with its associated increase in aggressive behavior, could compensate for a certain number of psychological problems, but if the hormone is decreased then impotence occurs. Simple loss of male hormone alone, however, in an adult male animal is not sufficient to completely eliminate sexual capacity. It has long been known that an adult man who has been castrated is still capable of an erection and sexual coupling. The women of Rome took full advantage of this fact and enjoyed themselves when they observed that their castrated slaves were still able to maintain an erection.

There are many causes for impotence. When age is not a factor, psychological reasons are perhaps the most common cause. However, there are numerous health conditions that can cause impotence and should be considered. Endocrine or hormone factors can be a cause of impotence, although often this is merely a contributory factor or it will decrease the frequency of sexual desire and sexual activity rather than causing a complete cessation of sexual capacity. Any severe medical illness can usually decrease a person's ability to engage in sexual activity. Diseases of the circulation can affect potency. The arteries that provide the blood supply to the penis can be obstructed by fatty deposits to the point that it is impossible to provide enough blood to the penis to maintain erection. This is sometimes associated with difficulty in walking because of insufficient blood supply to the legs. The older man who suffers from cramps in his legs when walking and from impotency is a recognized victim of fatty deposits in the arteries to the lower parts of his body.

Diseases which affect the nerves supplying the pelvic region can also cause impotence. High on the list of common diseases to induce such problems is diabetes. The diabetes may even be mild or relatively well controlled but because it affects the nerves to the pelvic region it can interfere with the normal function of the bladder and the ability to maintain an erection. Impotence is often one of the first signs of diabetes, and any man who has impotence should be examined for diabetes. Any disease which affects the nerves in this area, however, can cause impotence. A classic example of

155

this is the impotence that follows surgery in the pelvic region, such as removal of a rectal cancer. With some types of prostate operations, if the nerves are damaged or destroyed, the man will have impotence in the postoperative period. Sometimes this is transitory and function will return to normal. Disease of the prostate gland and infections will contribute to impotence in some individuals.

Because of the genuine distress that impotence causes both men and their wives, it is the source of a large number of letters from people worried by this problem.

Dear Dr. Lamb—I am twenty-one years of age and am finding myself no longer capable of achieving an erection. I have not experienced actual copulation. However, I am fully aware that I cannot get an erection. I may get one that will last perhaps only a few seconds, but as quickly as it comes it goes. I must confess that I have and do masturbate (something I cannot control), however, I do not achieve the hardness needed for copulation. This has me very worried as I would like to marry someday and have children, but I can't with this bothering me. If you can give me some suggestions and help I would appreciate it very much.

Comment—A young man with this type of problem needs a medical examination to be sure that there are no medical problems, and if there are none, he deserves counseling. Sometimes simple reassurance is all that is needed. Impotence in young men, particularly at the beginning of their active heterosexual life, is common. Their nervous system has to be conditioned to heterosexual responses.

One of the most important causes of impotence is lack of confidence or fear of failure. Such a high premium is placed on masculinity within our society that the possibility of sexual failure is a real threat. Once the individual thinks he may be inferior or unable to engage in sexual activity and loses confidence, then indeed he is incapable of performing sexually. There are many psychological factors which contribute to this problem. These are often young men who have been

156

given a lot of misinformation about the harmful effects of masturbation. Then, should they experience difficulty in sexual performance, they believe it's because of their masturbation. Other young men have a generalized overall feeling of guilt about sexual activity because of what they have been led to believe in their earlier development.

Dear Dr. Lamb—I have been unable during the past few months to sustain an erection to have sexual intercourse with my wife. I desire to have intercourse but am at an absolute loss as to why this happens. My wife doesn't understand either and it really puts me on the spot. She accuses me of having sex with someone else or not desiring her. I would deeply appreciate any help you could give me. I am thirty-one years old.

Comment—Provided there are no medical reasons, such a case may well illustrate another example of psychologically induced impotence. Impotence is not necessarily an indication that a man doesn't love his wife. It may also indicate he loves her too much. The classic Freudian concept in this circumstance is that the man is unable to reorganize his love concepts. In his early childhood his first deep sensuous love was with his mother, and because of the incest taboo, sexual relationships with this loved female were forbidden. When the adult male then loves a woman, he will find it difficult to have a sexual relationship with her because sexual activity was forbidden with his first loved woman, his mother.

Whether these theoretical considerations are always applicable or not, it is true that some men love their wife or sweetheart so much that they find it difficult to have satisfactory sexual relations. This is sometimes caused by the feeling that sexual activity is dirty or degrading. Many of these same men are fully capable of having sexual activity with a prostitute or a woman they consider socially inferior. This is one reason why some men find it necessary to degrade a woman before they can have sexual relations with her.

In other instances, which may well be the case here, the

man may be trying to achieve a performance record. He engages in sexual activity not out of desire but out of a need to measure up to a standard. Pressures created by this attempt to meet a certain performance level contribute to impotence. One of the best treatments for impotence is an understanding woman who does not pressure her partner for sex. A good technique is to enjoy physical intimacy with the understanding in advance that no sexual activity will take place. The lack of the need to perform removes the fear of failure and sometimes has surprising results.

Dear Dr. Lamb—I am forty-eight years old and have what my wife and I consider a very serious problem. I cannot get an erection. I have had this condition for two or three years and have been seeking medical help, to no avail.

I was married to my first wife for twenty-three years and during this marriage she became an alcoholic and turned frigid on me. For the last five years of this marriage, I was denied all sexual relations. We divorced, and I remarried. My present wife is everything the first one wasn't and we love each other dearly, but the problem persists. I have been to a doctor and he gave me a complete examination and massaged my prostate and studied my urine. Then he decided that I needed psychiatric help so he sent me to a psychiatrist. After several sessions, the psychiatrist sent me to a psychoanalyst and after two visits and a lot of money, I have given up. Do you have any suggestions?

Comment—Going to a psychiatrist was a very good idea and should have been continued. These problems are not always resolved in one or two visits, but may require several months, a year, or even longer in some instances. A very frequent psychological cause for impotence is a hostile marriage. This occurs when a couple actually hate each other but live together simply for convenience, social pressure, or most often, for financial reasons. The woman frequently is surprised when she can't arouse her husband sexually. In truth the level of hostility is so great that the man is unable to have the type of tender sentiments and emotional feelings that lead to satisfactory sexual relations.

Similarly, the wife may become frigid and refuse to respond to her husband's advances. Within the framework of the hostile marriage, sexual withholding by the wife is a frequent weapon. This is a particularly disastrous weapon if the man's moral characteristics prevent him from seeking a sexual outlet in other ways, specifically other women or masturbation. Apparently, sexual withholding occurred in this man's case with his first wife. Long-standing sexual disappointment and refusal can lead to fairly persistent impotence. It requires a period of time for such a man to work out his problem which usually requires professional counseling to achieve and return to a normal sex life.

Dear Dr. Lamb—My husband is in his early fifties and it is the second marriage for both of us. Our only problem is that he is impotent. In nearly two years of marriage we have had sex only six or eight times. Without going into more detail, is it possible for a man to be physically impotent and still have occasional wet dreams? I suspect this problem is a mental block because his first marriage and resultant divorce made him a woman-hater. The wife used sex as a means of getting things and was a very selfish person. She did a very good job of castrating him emotionally, but if wet dreams mean he is not physically impotent then I will try to get him to see a psychiatrist, which he has agreed he would eventually try.

Comment—Here is an example of a man who had difficulties with one marriage in which sexual withholding by the wife was used as a manipulative tool. The woman's choice of words in saying she had castrated him emotionally are quite accurate. Many such women fit the mold of what is called the castrating female.

This woman is also correct in her observation about wet dreams. If a man has erections on occasions other than when

159

sexual intercourse is attempted, he has proved that the body mechanisms are all intact and capable of producing an erection and that the real problem is in the brain or emotional mechanism. Nocturnal erections with wet dreams are a clear signal that this is true. This does not mean that this is a conscious failure on the part of the brain. It is beyond the control of the individual and that's why professional help is necessary.

Such individuals do not need hormones or medical attention of that type. What they need is professional counseling or psychiatric help. In such instances there is a high probability of success with adequate counseling, particularly when there is an understanding, sympathetic wife who can help work with the problem, which would seem to be the case as indicated by this woman's letter.

Incidentally, it should not be assumed that a man who has wet dreams is not obtaining sexual satisfaction. Men who have had sexual intercourse before going to sleep on occasions will have wet dreams. Nocturnal erections are the rule. This is merely one of the natural mechanisms of sexual responses. Some women fall into the trap of thinking that if their husband has a nocturnal erection, he is not getting full sexual satisfaction, and particularly if he happens to have a wet dream. This is not true. Some men are more likely to have wet dreams than others, with or without a completely satisfactory sexual life.

Dear Dr. Lamb—My husband is fifty-two and he has been impotent for over a year. Our doctor calls it a change of life. His erection is not very strong, and it fades, then vanishes once intercourse gets underway. What is the cause of this and what can be done to help cure it? He has been on a tranquilizer for about two years for a nervous stomach. Our marriage is beginning to go on the rocks. Where can we get some help?

Comment—Starting with the family doctor is a good place. Medical factors should be eliminated first. Certain drugs, including tranquilizers, can contribute to impotency. Any

160

medicine that is not definitely needed for a medical program should be discontinued to see whether or not it is contributing to the problem. This should be done under a doctor's supervision, however, since many medicines are absolutely essential to people and that's why they were prescribed in the first place.

Another cause for loss of erection during intercourse is the woman's anatomy. The middle-aged woman, particularly if she has had several children, may have a relaxed vaginal vault due to the stretching of muscles and ligaments with childbirth. There may not be enough muscular contraction around the loose vaginal vault to successfully hold the penis in place and provide adequate stimulation to the man. Instead the penis flops in and out with little or no friction. A woman with this problem should have the muscles in her pelvis and around the vagina tightened up, which can be done surgically. This form of surgical correction should be done in any woman with this problem anyway to correct or to prevent other difficulties that she can have with a fallen womb, fallen bladder, or even a rectum that is protruding into the vaginal vault.

Dear Dr. Lamb—Will heavy drinking cause a man to be impotent? My husband is in his latter thirties and he drinks four to five bottles of beer a day, which he says isn't heavy drinking. He shows signs of heavier drinking at other times. He is practically impotent. When I mention what this is doing to his sex life or his brain, he says I am preaching. I really need help.

Comment—Alcohol can cause impotence, particularly if used in large quantities. Masters and Johnson report that alcohol is a major cause of impotency in American men. Considerable variation exists, however. A small amount of alcohol can actually relieve inhibitions and stimulate some people to sexual activity. Even modest amounts of alcohol in other individuals can have an inhibiting effect on their sexual capacity.

Dear Dr. Lamb—My husband is a handsome, energetic,

161

ambitious forty-three-year-old man. He is also nervous, anxious, and an alcoholic. He has been going to AA for a couple of years and stayed sober with one exception, I think, all that time. He has never been an affectionate person, and for many years I felt my love was one-sided but that he needed me. He was always very passionate, though, and we had a very satisfactory sex life.

For the past six months, his passion is nonexistent and our sex life has dwindled in quantity and about two months ago it suffered in quality. I feel he does it just to please me, but it is not much better than nothing. He doesn't seem to be fully stimulated.

One time not long ago he came in early in the morning from a trip out of town and he had been drinking. He was his old passionate self and it was delightful. He has never admitted that he had been drinking, but later on he said that if he ever started drinking again it would be to regain his sexual drive. It would be terrible to have him drunk again, but this thing between us is terrible too. Could it be that this is mental and only temporary? If it's physical, is there anything that can be done?

Comment—If this lady's observations are correct, it would seem that alcohol releases this individual's inhibitions. Both excessive use of alcohol and impotence are frequently caused by psychiatric problems, which may be mild or severe. Impotence after stopping alcohol suggests psychological factors are important. After a complete medical examination I should think such a person deserves good psychiatric treatment, both for the problem of alcohol and the problem of impotence.

Dear Dr. Lamb—We have had some bad experience with the side effects of a drug my husband took for high cholesterol, and it made him impotent. Is this common?

Comment—There are a number of medicines that cause impotence. These include certain medicines for the treatment of high blood pressure and heart disease. Because impotence is so common, however, it should not be assumed that it's caused by medicine that a person is taking unless that fact is established. The best way to do this is for the doctor to discontinue the medicines and see if the problem is alleviated.

Some medicines are well known for this effect. They are principally those which block the nerves which control contractions of the arteries. These medicines are used in treatment of high blood pressure. Some of the other medicines used in treatment of high blood pressure can affect the man's ability to have an orgasm, although they do not affect the man's ability to obtain an erection. Some tranquilizers can also have this effect.

Dear Dr. Lamb—About two years ago I had the Asiatic flu and just preceding this I had been on a diet and lost about thirty pounds. I was taking vitamin pills and my supply ran out and I took some from another bottle which I thought were One-A-Day, but they proved to be female hormones. The grandchildren had destroyed the label. I lost my manhood for some reason, and I cannot get an erection. Did these female hormones cause this, and how long do they hold on? Is there any correction for it? I am past sixty but did not have this condition previous to this time. My family doctor brings up age when I ask him about this.

Comment—Rapid weight loss can sometimes cause impotency. In other instances it will decrease the ability to have an orgasm, although the man can still sustain an erection. In general, poor nutrition contributes to a decrease in sex drive and can cause impotence. Administration of female hormones, if given in sufficient amounts over a period of time, can cause femininization of a man, including large breasts and loss of sex drive. This problem disappears shortly after the female hormones are withdrawn and a normal hormone balance is achieved.

Failure to perform for any reason can raise doubt in a man's mind and then you have compounded the problem

163

with fear of failure. There seem to be quite a number of men in their latter forties, fifties, and early sixties who experience impotence. Nevertheless I am not in sympathy with the common practice of doctors to merely pass this off as just being old enough to "forget about sex." This advice is more often given by younger physicians than older physicians in the same age group. A complete examination including measurement of the amount of male hormone that is present is indicated. Certainly in a large number of men who are only sixty years of age or younger, there are things which can be done to help improve their sexual capacity, if they are having persistent impotence.

Dear Dr. Lamb—I have read that testosterone is very effective in the treatment of impotency in men over fifty, when it's just a matter of age. Is this true? If so, are there any undesirable side effects?

Comment—Yes, testosterone is useful in individuals who have low testosterone levels. It is of no benefit in men who do not have a definite decrease in testosterone. A number of men have a gradual decrease in the amount of testosterone that is produced, and the male-female hormone balance is reversed. As I mentioned earlier, this may well be related to fatty deposits in the arteries. To prevent fatty deposits in the arteries that supply blood to the testicles, one should follow the same program advocated to prevent fatty deposits to arteries that cause heart attacks and strokes.

Testosterone given to younger men who have normal hormone functions may actually inhibit the testicle's ability to form sperm. Therefore, it is not a panacea or treatment for all forms of impotence.

Some men benefit from getting testosterone because of its placebo effect. They are told the pill will help their nature and they believe they will be potent. Therefore, it improves their confidence. Whenever they have regained their confidence, they are apt to be able to return to normal sexual function. If this confidence is achieved through the bark of an African tree, testosterone, or sugar pill, it makes no difference. The confidence is what restores the potency.

Dear Dr. Lamb—About two years ago I had one testicle removed because of cancer. I got along fine and have never had any trouble since. However, I have never been able to have intercourse since the operation, even though I still have one testicle. My doctor has given me hormone pills but so far, no good. Do you believe it would be safe for me to take some of the more effective drugs like Spanish fly, for example, or should I call it quits? When I did try intercourse on two occasions, there was no discharge whatever. I have never had any prostate trouble and wonder why there shouldn't be any discharge of any kind. I am sixty-two years of age.

Comment—Loss of one testicle by itself is not sufficient cause for impotence. Commonly individuals with only one testicle have a normal sexual drive and are able to perform normally with no problem of impotence. Therefore, the difficulty here must be something else. In this man's age group the loss of a testicle, however, might really contribute to the decreased available male hormone (testosterone) for the body.

The discharge of an orgasm is not dependent on the testicles. They only produce the sperm cell which constitutes a very small part of the volume of an orgasm. Most of the fluid comes from the seminal vesicle and prostate gland. The function of these structures, however, is dependent upon the presence of sufficient amounts of testosterone.

Spanish fly has proved to be an effective aphrodisiac but it does so by causing inflammation of the urethra. It's also a poison which, if taken in too large a quantity, can cause death. Its physical composition is ground beetle, a particular type of insect found in southern Europe. There are large lists of substances that have been recommended for the treatment of impotence. Most of them are totally ineffective. Others are downright dangerous. Men suffering from impotence are easy victims for charlatans. I would strongly advise against

165

the use of any medications or treatments unless under a doctor's advice. In those cases that are truly caused by low testosterone levels some aid can be obtained by administering male hormones. As an example of the long-term myths of taking different substances for impotence, Dr. Thomas Benedek of the University of Pittsburgh School of Medicine cited Maimonides (1135-1204) recommended potion for the treatment of impotency: "Take the penis of an ox, dry it and grind it. Sprinkle some of this on a soft-boiled egg, and drink it in sips." There are numerous other remedies that have been advocated which are equally ridiculous.

Dear Dr. Lamb—My problem is I lack sex drive. I am sixty-five years old, and in the last year I seem to be slipping. I have no erection. Everything else is normal. Is there any help for me, such as a transplant or other treatment? My doctor has given me some hormones which helped me a little.

Comment—Whether the hormones merely restored the man's confidence or really replaced a deficiency of male hormone cannot be known without objective information from laboratory measurements. Transplants aren't the answer for impotence. It's not very likely that you can transplant an erect penis, and transplanting testicles, if a successful operation were feasible, would provide only a momentary increase in male hormone. There is no indication for transplants for impotence.

Dear Dr. Lamb—I am seventy-six years old, well-built, vigorous, and healthy. Impotence is my only problem. Is there anything that can be done? I have had a few wet dreams and there's plenty of sperm, but I don't seem to respond. Is this a disease? Would transplantation of goat gland help?

Comment—Shades of Dr. Brinkley, the famous quack and charlatan who grafted pieces of goat gland into the testicles of many gullible and hopeful men! While there may have been some momentary benefit from the hormone in the

166

grafted glands, this would soon be exhausted. In most instances grafts of this sort wouldn't even be tolerated by the body, but would be rejected, thereby leaving the testicles that had received the wedge implant of goat testicle more damaged than before.

Having a nocturnal emission or wet dream suggests that a man is still potent. However, a person who is not able to obtain an erection can still have a nocturnal emission. That is, the fluid flows out of the flaccid penis during sleep. Thus, to be certain that a wet dream really means that a man has retained his physical ability for sexual intercourse, it must be known that the penis is actually erected at the time of the wet dream.

About 50 percent of the men in this man's age group do have problems with impotence. In our society it is accepted as a normal consequence of aging. This does not mean that it's not preventable. It means that very little has actually been done about the problem.

Dear Dr. Lamb—I am twenty-four years old and engaged to a man in his latter thirties. We plan to be married soon. His wife died five years ago, and he has no children. Despite the difference in our age, we communicate well and are very much in love. Three years ago he was cured of a drinking problem and hasn't drunk since then. I have never had intercourse, but he has never even attempted to seduce me. Because of my own beliefs about premarital sex I have not attempted to seduce him. Sex hasn't been any part of our relationship. Doctor, is it possible that he is impotent? If so, what's the cure for alcoholic impotency?

Please help me. I have waited so long for the man I love and I now fear for our wedding night as well as the nights that follow.

Comment—It is dangerous for a woman to jump to premature conclusions. If a woman is suspicious of her man's sexual capacity, she will convey, one way or another, her doubts and fears. This in itself may cause her man to be insecure,

167

lack confidence, and therefore be impotent. Never underestimate the fact that the sex act is a confidence game as much as anything else. Both partners should attempt to build up each other's egos. Destructive attitudes and suspicions do very little to accomplish this goal. It is advisable, however, for couples who are anticipating marriage to have at least discussed sex and sexual attitudes prior to the wedding ceremony. This can also help to reduce a lot of anxiety. The intimacy of courtship and engagement serves a genuine purpose.

PREMATURE EJACULATION

Dear Dr. Lamb—I am twenty-four years old and my problem is that all of my adult life I have been experiencing premature ejaculation. It has gotten to the point where my wife is asking for a divorce. Can you tell me what causes this? Could this be cured by surgery or is there some other type of medical treatment for it?

Comment—Premature ejaculation occurs in young people and is thought by some individuals to be an example of strong sex drive. Most instances of premature ejaculation can be helped or cured by conditioning techniques of the type recommended by Masters and Johnson. Men with this problem are usually overly excited. They have become conditioned to respond rapidly to sexual stimulation. The sexual response is quick, it builds to a peak level, and the show is over. The real problem, exemplified by this young man's letter, is that as soon as the man has an orgasm he is then temporarily normally impotent and unable to sexually satisfy his wife. With each recurring experience, excitement builds to a peak quickly and the same problem occurs.

Much of the Masters and Johnson technique for treating many sexual problems is directed toward getting away from the necessity to perform, or the sexual obstacle course, and learning to relax in a sexual atmosphere with a member of the opposite sex. This is accomplished by prohibiting sexual activity at the beginning of the treatment. The couple lie

168

together in the nude, learn to stroke each other and express affection for each other without stimulating each other's genitals or engaging in sexual activity. After several days of relaxed affectionate activity without the necessity of sexual performance, many anxieties and nervous reactions are decreased or removed.

In addition, reflex mechanisms can be helpful in preventing premature ejaculation. As the man nears the point of orgasm, the head of the penis is squeezed on the underneath surface until the sexual tension subsides. This is done by placing the thumb under the head of the penis where it joins the shaft and two fingers over the opposite side and squeezing firmly. By repeating this over and over, after a period of time, the man becomes conditioned to being sexually aroused without reaching the peak of orgasm. After he has been conditioned to this type of response, which in these individuals must be a learned response, he is able to prolong his period of sexual excitement and proceed to normal sexual relations. After the squeeze method has been perfected and orgasm delayed, then the man can gently insert his penis without making any thrusting movements and get used to this condition without rising to the height of excitement that precipitates an orgasm.

This technique appears to be more successful than attempts to anesthetize the head of the penis with medications or other procedures which have been suggested. One of the main achievements of the conditioning and squeeze technique is to relieve excessive sexual tensions which actually inhibit sexual performance. Since many men achieve premature ejaculation just at the time of entrance into the vagina or at the very onset of physical sexual contact, it is clear that they have an overactive reflex mechanism stimulated by their emotional and mental responses. This is why the conditioning approach combined with the squeeze technique is useful.

Dear Dr. Lamb—My husband has asked me to write about our problem. We have been married over thirty years

169

and have had very little sex life. Our problem is that we are Catholic and can't use many forms of birth control, and when I've been pregnant, because I'm prone to having miscarriages, our doctor has limited our sexual activity.

We used the rhythm method as a means of birth control, but despite this we have had four children. Combined with the problems of my pregnancy and the rhythm method, we haven't had much intercourse, and more recently I have had radiation therapy of my uterus. Now there's no danger of pregnancy, but my husband is not capable of the marriage act for more than a minute. We cannot touch each other as he would have a discharge very quickly. He gets relief for his discharge and I just get to feeling as a disposal unit. We love each other and feel helpless. We went to our family doctor and he was unable to help. We wondered if there is anything new in the line of medicine that would be available.

Comment—The circumstances this woman describes certainly are not conducive to developing a mature, relaxed sexual relationship. The letter points out that even after years of marriage, a man who is having difficulty with premature ejaculation can continue to be plagued with the problem. Conditioning exercises of the type I have discussed are perhaps the best approach. Some individuals benefit from psychotherapy if they truly have a basic underlying psychological problem, but sometimes the conditioning and squeeze technique recommended by Masters and Johnson is the most rapid approach to correcting this problem in performance.

A variation to the squeeze technique is to provide sexual stimulation, usually manually, up to the point of orgasm and then stop all form of sexual stimulation. By repeatedly doing this the male becomes conditioned to being sexually aroused up to the point of orgasm without actually having one. This slows down his overall sexual response and accustoms him to a more prolonged form of activity. These conditioning exercises, whether it is the squeeze technique or masturbation,

170

are best carried out with the sexual partner. The sexual partner should do the squeezing and participate in the sexual stimulation.

ORGASM FAILURE

Dear Dr. Lamb—I am recently married and have encountered a revelation which has shocked me and I cannot get an explanation from my husband other than "I was born that way." Our sexual relationship appears to be normal in all ways, but there is no orgasm whatever from my husband or moisture of any kind. In the beginning I thought perhaps he was suppressing release to avoid pregnancy, and this is what he led me to believe. Now I know this is not the case. Please tell me what is wrong. Is this what is known as a vasectomy? Is he normal? How can we have satisfactory fulfillment this way? I am worried and this situation is beginning to affect my relationship with him. He appears satisfied, but I am beginning to believe it is a cover-up. Is this an abnormality? Please, doctor, I need your help.

Comment—This is an uncommon form of sexual failure. It is completely unsatisfactory for the man, but it can provide adequate stimulation for the woman. It interferes with the female's enjoyment of sex from two standpoints. Occasionally men with this problem continue or repeat intercourse so frequently that their wives complain. No matter how frequent or how long the thrusting is continued, the man fails to have an orgasm. The other complaint from the woman is that she feels a need to recognize her mate's sexual satisfaction. If he is not satisfied in his sexual relations, she feels that something is lacking in herself, just as a man often feels it's his fault if the woman doesn't achieve orgasm. (Sometimes it is his fault, and in other instances it's the woman's attitude.)

In this condition, everything is intact and working normally. What's really occurring is a form of psychological block.

171

Professional counseling is reported to be highly successful in most individuals with this problem. Some can solve their own problem by experimentation and being honest with each other. A man may know what will trigger an orgasm. If he communicates freely with his sexual partner and tells her what "turns him on," she may be able to provide the appropriate stimulus and once he has broken the orgasm barrier, their relationship may improve rapidly.

IX

Female Sexual Dysfunction

WOMEN AS WELL AS MEN may have a sexual dysfunction. The inability of the woman to respond sexually is sometimes called frigidity. This term, however, has very little meaning and many sexologists prefer not to use it. For this reason, the more inclusive phrase "female sexual dysfunction" is used here.

The large number of letters that relate to these problems essentially encompasses three categories: lack of sexual desire or sexual interest, difficulty in reaching an orgasm, and painful intercourse, called dyspareunia.

LACK OF DESIRE

There are many reasons why a woman loses all interest in sexual activity. To discover the underlying factors requires careful interviewing and evaluation of the individual situation. Lack of sexual desire can be a source of considerable stress to both the man and the woman. It should be emphasized that whenever there is sexual dysfunction in either the male or the female, both partners are really having a sexual problem. When a woman loses her desire for sex, it inevitably affects the sexual behavior of the male. One man's description of his problem, resulting from such a situation, is as follows:

173

Dear Dr. Lamb—My wife and I are fifty years old and have a problem, and I wish you would put my mind at ease. The problem has existed for many years. Over ten years ago my wife had a hysterectomy, including the removal of both ovaries. Since that time we have had no sex life at all. She declares she has no feelings at all in regards to sex, saying it is impossible due to the removal of her ovaries, etc. I had spoken to her doctor before surgery and was assured she would have a better sex life after surgery than before. I have spoken to others who have had the same operation my wife has had, and they have informed me that they have had no problems whatsoever. Having spoken to her doctor about our problem, he informed me her problem was more in her mind and that she could have been helped but she must ask for help and she has always refused to do this, saying it concerned us and no one else.

We do not sleep in the same room any more. I keep away from the temptation of needing her. This has done my health no good. I have been under the care of my own doctor for nerves brought about by frustration and so forth. He has put me in the hospital a number of times and gotten me back in fairly good health only to go down in health within a few days after I have gone home. I have never in all these years been with another woman. I have spoken to my minister and family services, but my wife has never asked for help and has refused to do so.

She is cold toward her sons and me. She never shows any affection. We do not quarrel, we just endure each other. We are quite comfortable in material things, no debts, we have money and a good home. I have a good position, and we have everything but we are poor in love and affection. Our marriage has little meaning and exists in name only. I feel like taking my doctor's advice and just leaving home, for it means nothing any more.

If I have judged my wife unfairly, please say so. I

have got to the point now in life where I need help. I have no bad habits, do not drink, or go out and leave her alone. Now I do not sleep very well and have a lot of stomach trouble. My doctor tells me this is mostly nerves and frustration. I need an outside opinion. Would you be kind enough to help me. The type of life I have had to live these years has been far from pleasant, to say the least.

Comment—Considering that the woman is now fifty years of age, she must have had her surgery before she reached forty. Very often, female hormone replacement is indicated after surgical removal of both ovaries. Without adequate amounts of female hormone, a woman will lose her interest in sex and in general her female sex organs will "dry up." Her external sex organs become smaller, and the vaginal vault will become dry and small, particularly if sexual activity is not maintained regularly. With the small, dry vaginal vault, sexual intercourse is painful. A surgical procedure which removes the ovaries at an early age essentially puts the woman into a premature menopause.

The first step in resolving this problem is a complete medical examination of the wife to see if indeed she needs hormone therapy. This could enable her to have the normal female secretions in the vagina, eliminating the dryness and protecting her from painful intercourse. It might also increase her sexual responsiveness. If there are other underlying factors, which would be psychological in nature, they would need to be explored, identified, and dealt with. It is certainly not normal for a woman before the age of forty to discontinue having any interest in sex and withdraw totally from her husband and sons.

It is important to emphasize that women who have a hysterectomy and have their ovaries still in place do not have this problem. As long as the ovaries are functioning and producing normal amounts of female hormone, the normal function of the vagina and female organs continues and the operation should in no way interfere with continued normal sexual activity.

175

When a woman practices sexual withholding within the marriage, it is particularly difficult for the man whose personal morality prevents him from relieving his sexual tensions by finding another woman or engaging in masturbation. The accumulated sexual tensions will indeed take their toll in increased nervousness and irritability. The entire situation is potentially emotionally injurious and can also produce physical problems including stomach disorders and insomnia. It can further lead to a decrease in sexual capacity of the male, if the practice is continued for long periods of time.

Dear Dr. Lamb—I am thirty years of age, have two small children and a wonderful patient husband. My problem is I have no desire for sexual intercourse. Maybe once or twice a month I really want to have intercourse. The rest of the time I try to avoid it. This lack of marital love is very hard on my husband. I love him very much and promise myself that I'll not disappoint him any more. Needless to say, I continue to say no. We cannot afford my going to a psychiatrist, but something has to be done. Is there some kind of hormone I could take to increase my sex drive?

Comment—Women have different levels of frequency for sexual desire just as do men. Some women actually just aren't interested in having sex frequently. Others want it every day. The difficulty occurs when a woman who doesn't care for sex very often is married to a man who wants it frequently, or vice versa. The fact that this woman says she would like to have intercourse once or twice a month indicates that from time to time she does enjoy normal sexual activity. It is only the frequency that is a problem.

This kind of difficulty should be clearly discussed by the two, and she should make a real effort on her part to satisfy his sexual needs, even though it may not always be necessary or desirable for her. If she loves him strongly, as her letter indicates, her desire to please him should be adequate reason for sex. In the long run she may be surprised to find out she

176

is enjoying it more since successful sexual relations build on each other and reinforce the sexual pattern and sexual response.

Dear Dr. Lamb—I am in my mid-fifties and healthy. We had a good marriage until my husband, through too much social drinking, became an alcoholic. He has stopped drinking, but I find that I am "turned off" sexually and unable to respond. He accuses me of having a lover, which is ridiculous. I love my husband very much really. I think it was those years when I was so filled with resentment toward him for what he was doing to me and to our children that have done this to me. Is this likely? I would like very much to be a "normal" and loving wife again and to please my husband.

Comment—One of the first requirements for a woman to have sexual desire for her husband and respond appropriately is that she respect and love her husband. This woman says she loves her husband, but there was a period in which, her letter states frankly, she resented him. When a woman loses her respect for a man, it often shows up in their sexual relationship. Even after the husband has "reformed," the experience of the resentment remains, and the image of the man as he was leaves a permanent blur on his image as a knight in shining armor and a lover. Unfortunately, after having an ideal shattered, some women have difficulty in returning to a normal pleasurable sexual relationship.

Sometimes if the couple takes a vacation away from their surroundings and the events that created the difficulty, as well as their children, they can gain a new lease on their sex life. It also helps to talk it out with each other, as long as this is talking and not arguing, accusing, or otherwise punishing each other.

A modified Masters and Johnson technique will sometimes help. This means having periods of intimacy and petting together which eliminates, by prior agreement, sexual activity. Over a period of several days the couple will learn what kinds of activity stimulate their partner. Gradually, they increase their intimacy until intercourse is pleasurable to each.

Dear Dr. Lamb—I have a problem which has been bothering me for a long time, and that is whether or not a person can be allergic to another person with whom he quite frequently comes in contact. What would cause a wife to break out in an itching, burning rash whenever her husband approaches her sexually or otherwise, especially if he has been drinking heavily? I am ashamed to discuss this with my doctor for fear he will think I am some sort of freak. It does seem rather silly other than the fact I simply cannot tolerate people who drink to excess. Won't you please say something about this unique affliction?

Comment—Hives and rashes are ofttimes a sign of emotional stress. This woman's observation that she is "allergic" to her husband is probably correct. The rash is an emotional response to her fear and hostility toward her husband when he has been drinking. There are no small number of women who find sexual relations with a drunken husband distasteful. Some women state that they feel like a prostitute when their husband is "using them" under the influence of alcohol. These responses also indicate the large amount of negative thoughts that have been programmed into the woman's mind, probably from childhood, about sex.

Dear Dr. Lamb—I am writing you as I have a problem which I am sure many other people have. To begin with, it's all about sex, and I have been married thirty years. My husband and I have fourteen kids, and right now I am forty-eight years old and my problem seems to be that I am just fed up with having anything to do with sex. All my husband and I do is argue. He keeps telling me I don't care to keep him happy any more. Sometimes I try to be with him, but at the same time, I just give up. I really don't know if it's because I'm

178

always sick or because of my age. What do you think is the problem?

Comment—There are probably fourteen reasons for this woman's loss of interest in sex—all of them kids. Any woman who has to look after fourteen children obviously has a considerable load. Just as the man who is over-involved in his work can lose interest in sex, so can a woman. If she is kept busy by a large number of children or by the multiple activities of even fewer children, or by social commitments, she too can lose interest in sex. It is all she can do to manage her daily affairs, without the added complication of sex. Arguments and hostilities between husbands and wives can often lead to a loss of interest in sex. The disinterest is not the cause of the problem, but a symptom.

Dear Dr. Lamb—I am a woman of thirty and although I have never had a lot of sex drive, I seem to have less as I get older. My husband is a wonderful person and provider. He has a lot of sex drive. My doctor tells me there is nothing wrong with me so far as vitamins or disorders go. I don't have the nerve to ask him if he has some kind of shots he could give me. I believe there are hormone shots. Could you advise me what other women do in a situation like this? My husband would really be pleased if I'd start and respond to sex a lot more than I do.

Comment—This situation would require considerable exploring to find out just what is causing this woman's difficulty. Her observation that her husband would really be pleased if she improved her sexual performance is probably accurate. Most men are more likely to feel that they have been successful sexually if their wives have responded to them. If the wife doesn't respond they are apt to feel that they have been inadequate as a lover. Sometimes this is true, but in other instances it lies in psychological factors within the woman beyond the control of her sexual partner. The real reasons may lie in childhood orientations on sexual matters, such as the belief in childhood that sex is dirty or wicked or immoral.

ORGASM FAILURE

Theoretically, all women should be able to have an orgasm. There are a lot of misconceptions about the orgasm itself. It is not necessary for a woman to have an orgasm to enjoy sex, and it is not necessary for a woman to have an orgasm to get pregnant. Surveys of women's response to masturbation report that most women do not experience orgasms until their latter teens, even though they may have been manipulating and stimulating themselves for several years prior to the first experienced orgasm. Despite the fact that apparently every woman should be able to have an orgasm, Dr. Philip Polatin, psychiatrist at Columbia University, states that the general concensus is that female orgasms occur in about 60 to 70 percent of married women usually or always and 25 percent of them have orgasms "some of the time," while 5 to 10 percent have orgasms rarely or never.

There has long been much confusion over the nature of the female orgasm. At one time it was thought there was a difference between an orgasm associated with the clitoris and an orgasm associated with the vagina. Much was made about the psychiatric significance of whether a woman had a clitoral orgasm or a vaginal orgasm. This Freudian fallacy was laid to rest when the experimental observations of Masters and Johnson demonstrated photographically in the laboratory what the female orgasm is. It was conclusively established that a woman has neither a clitoral nor a vaginal orgasm but a total orgasmic response which involves all of the female genital system and even the breasts. The stages of sexual arousal, response, orgasm, and remission are essentially the same in a woman as they are in a male except of course that the male's ejaculation is unique.

The woman's genitals become congested with blood during sexual excitement and undergo color changes. The breasts undergo changes in size and reaction throughout the sexual experience to the point of orgasm. The breast changes aren't as noticeable in a woman who has nursed children, since this will affect the vascularity, tendons, and other structures within the breasts. This, however, doesn't lessen a woman's sexual pleasure.

Dear Dr. Lamb—I have been married for nine years and I have two lovely children. I am twenty-nine and have never reached a climax in my entire life. Some women may be satisfied knowing this is normal for them, but I am not. What I would like to know is what causes women to behave this way, and has science come up with some solution to help women overcome this hold-back? I think it would worry me to death to go through life and not know how it really feels to reach a climax.

Comment—There are many reasons why some women never experience a climax. No doubt a large part of this is related to the type of sexual training they had as children. A negative attitude toward sex throughout childhood is usually more inhibiting to the female than it is to the male. Religious prohibitions are more often directed at the girl than at the boy. The girl often simply doesn't learn to appreciate sex and is unable to overcome all of these negative feelings.

This problem is compounded if she is unable to identify with her sexual partner, and there are many reasons why identification might not be successful. For a woman to have an orgasm, she must indeed give herself to her sexual partner.

Many different sources of fear enter into the problem, too, including fear of pregnancy and fear of venereal disease, and before sex is experienced, fear of sexual activity itself. A great deal can be done to help women who have not had an orgasm. Masters and Johnson report success in about four out of five cases. Although their method is lengthier and more complex than can be reported here, the chief goal is to examine the relationship, neutralize or limit negative feelings that may exist, and then introduce the couple into a situation of physical intimacy short of intercourse. Prohibiting intercourse in the early stages of the treatment removes the necessity to perform and enables the couple to merely learn to communicate with each other physically.

After the initial efforts, depending on the speed of progress, the art of stimulation can be improved. This means that the woman has to relax some of her inhibitions and teach her mate what stimulates her the most in the petting situation. When the husband discovers what the woman's actual preferences are, he can apply these in their sexual relations. Some women are turned off sexually because the husband manipulates the head of the clitoris, which is unusually sensitive and dry at the beginning of sex play. This can cause pain and irritation. It also can lead to premature excitement before the rest of the woman's sexual response is turned on. In the early sexual response, the woman needs to secrete fluids from the wall of the vagina which serve as nature's lubricant for the sexual act.

From there on, the next phase of the Masters and Johnson technique is based mostly on allowing the woman to take the initiative, and gradually learning to enjoy the sex act.

Women who have never had an orgasm from any form of sexual stimulation, including masturbation, are relatively rare. Most psychiatrists feel that these women have an unusually strong history of inhibition and repressive influences in their early formative years. Dr. Donald Hastings, professor of psychiatry at the University of Minnesota, writing about this problem, describes the technique of overcoming the difficulty which he states he learned from married women. Put simply, the woman uses whatever device arouses her sexual interest the most, perhaps reading sexual literature, and having stimulated herself through this means then she manually stimulates herself, or in short, masturbates to the point of orgasm. This may take some time, but with repeated attempts she is usually able to do it. Once an orgasm has been achieved, even through masturbation, by repeated efforts the response is strengthened and can carry over into the marital relationship. Often the transfer can be made by having the husband do the manual stimulation for her before moving on to intercourse. Using similar techniques, some women have trained themselves to have multiple orgasms. This is compatible with the concept that masturbation prepares a woman for normal adult heterosexual activity.

Dear Dr. Lamb—I am twenty-six and have been pregnant before, fortunately I had a miscarriage. I want to know if there is anything physically wrong with me or if I am frigid, because I have never reached an orgasm or climax.

I am not married. I can't seem to relax when having intercourse. I am always afraid I might become pregnant. I was always taught that sex was wrong before marriage. I am not a bad person, but everybody is having sex these days. I think it's wrong to have sex before being married. Could that be the reason I can't reach a climax? I would also like to know if a person could get pregnant right after her menstrual period by not using any birth control measures? You see, I don't use birth control.

Comment—This letter contains many clues concerning why this woman fails to have an orgasm. It indicates a repressive and negative attitude about sex in her early developmental years. Morally, she thinks sex is wrong outside of wedlock, and very probably feels guilty because she is engaging in sex. This guilt, combined with a negative input about sex, in itself is sufficient to prevent some women from having a climax. Then combine that with her fear of pregnancy since she's single and particularly since she's been pregnant once before, and the situation is compounded. Finally, realize that she is not using birth control measures which should give her good cause to worry about the possibility of becoming pregnant. A woman can get pregnant right after her menstrual period since women are not always regular.

This woman should see a physician if for no other reason

than to obtain counseling about normal sex life and discuss whether or not she should be using birth control procedures. If she can dispel the guilt she feels about sex, there is a good probability that she will be able to have a normal sex life with orgasms.

Dear Dr. Lamb—I am twenty years old and I have been married less than a year. My problem is that I am unable to have a climax through intercourse. There is nothing wrong with my husband, and we are happy together. I have pretended to my husband that everything was normal. I thought the problem would go away after a while, but it hasn't and I'm getting worried. Many times I have thought about talking to my doctor, but I am too embarrassed. What could be physically wrong to cause this? Also, what could be done if my worrying about my inability has caused it to become something mental as well as physical? I need your advice.

Comment—This girl has the insight to realize that worrying about the problem may, indeed, be aggravating the situation. The first step is being honest with her husband. Sexual partners can't do much about improving their sexual performance and resolving their sexual difficulties unless they are willing to communicate with each other. In something that's so important to each individual, there's no reason that two individuals who are close enough to each other to be experiencing sexual intercourse shouldn't be able to discuss their responses with each other. Once the wife has acknowledged to her husband that a problem exists, they might try the modified Masters and Johnson technique which has been outlined in answers to previous questions.

Women who have not had orgasms at the beginning of their active sex life ofttimes do later. As they get older they relax more about their sexual activity, and if they are uninhibited enough to experiment a bit with their sexual partner, they can find new ways to stimulate themselves and increase their enjoyment of sexual activity. Just relaxing to a sex life

184

without expecting too much often does miracles, and in the course of several years the woman may suddenly begin to have orgasms. The following letter illustrates this point:

Dear Dr. Lamb—My husband and I have been very happily married for more than four years now, and we also wanted to have children soon after we were married. After we tried for about two months and hadn't been successful, I became worried that I was sterile because I was unable to have a sexual climax. Then, lo and behold, the following month I found out I was pregnant.

Two years after the first child was born, we had another one and still I had not had a climax. I became worried that I would never have one and wanting to give myself to my husband as completely as he gave himself to me, I consulted three doctors. They all said it was nothing to worry about as long as we both enjoyed intercourse. I even bought and read a copy of *The Sensuous Woman,* hoping that that would give me a clue as to why I was what I thought I was—an incomplete woman.

Then one night after we had been married more than three and a half years and I had given up all hope, it finally happened, so faintly that my husband had to tell me that it had actually occurred. After that it came more and more frequently and with increasing strength until now it is no effort at all to achieve a climax as many as four or five times in one half-hour period of intercourse.

Comment—This woman gradually conditioned herself to the point that she was having an orgasm. Remember that even though girls begin masturbation early in life, most of them don't experience orgasms until their latter teens, even though they may enjoy sexual experience.

A feeling of confidence and enjoyment on the part of the woman is just as essential to her having an orgasm as confidence is for the man to obtain an erection. One of the

185

beautiful things that this woman's husband did for her was to build up her confidence initially. Her description of her first orgasm raises a serious question as to whether she really had one or not, but by reassuring her, her husband helped build up her confidence. In this state her sexuality increased and gradually led to her ability to have several orgasms in succession. In short, she learned how to enjoy sex, which no doubt greatly improved her husband's sex life as well and improved their marriage.

Dear Dr. Lamb—I read in your column that male diabetics were sometimes impotent. What about the female diabetic? Does she have difficulty having orgasms? I am a forty-three-year-old diabetic and have had diabetes for thirty years and am in good health. Yet I have a very difficult time in having orgasms. Unfortunately my husband has not been a skillful lover. However, over the past several years I have studied the subject in detail and though we have improved our lovemaking abilities, I still cannot obtain an orgasm most of the time. I am disturbed about this lack.

Comment—That's a good question for there are a number of organic diseases which can cause the woman difficulty in having an orgasm. Nevertheless in the vast majority of women, failure to have an orgasm is based on psychological factors or lack of conditioning and proper sexual experience. In commenting specifically on the relationship of diabetes to the female orgasm, Dr. Robert Kolodny of Harvard Medical School reported that 44 out of 125 diabetic women had complete absence of an orgasm during the preceding year, whereas in a control group of 100 nondiabetic women only 6 of them had orgasmic failure. In other words about 35 percent of the women with diabetes had orgasmic failure compared to 6 percent of the women without diabetes. This strongly suggests that diabetes can be a factor in preventing a woman from obtaining an orgasm.

Dear Dr. Lamb—Please help me if you can. I am a married

186

man and have a lovely daughter, aged two years. Up until a short time ago my wife and I were still enjoying our sex life. I am thirty-five and she is thirty. She still satisfies my needs, but it seems I can't satisfy her anymore. I truly love her and say this with all my heart, but I am afraid our love life is going down the drain. In the name of God, please tell me what to do if you can.

Comment—I include this letter to show you the desperation that a man can feel when his wife is unable to respond sexually. This letter speaks eloquently for the fact that this type of response by the woman has a drastic effect on the man.

PAINFUL INTERCOURSE

Painful intercourse, or dyspareunia, precludes satisfactory sexual relationships. While it is true sometimes that painful intercourse masks a psychological problem, it is equally true that it can be caused by a disease or medical problem. If a woman has intercourse before she has started secreting sufficient amounts of vaginal lubricant, the relatively dry vaginal vault will be irritated during the sex act and cause pain. Inflammations of the vaginal vault from various infections can also cause pain. Injuries caused during birth or traumatic sexual experiences, such as rape, can cause painful intercourse. Dr. Robert L. Dickinson, commenting on this problem in *Human Sex Anatomy,* stated that in 161 women with painful intercourse, he found a physical reason for the difficulty in 118. Clearly this justifies a careful gynecological examination in any woman who complains of painful intercourse before assuming that her problem is "psychological."

Sometimes the female urethra is irritated by pressure of the erect penis trapping the urethra against the pubic bone. To help guard against this problem Dr. Dickinson suggested trying a different position, specifically elevating the woman's pelvis by use of a pillow and then avoiding pressure with the penis against the bony pubis during the sex act.

Dear Dr. Lamb—I had a baby four months ago. Since then my husband and I have not been able to have intercourse. It hurts me when he enters and withdraws. Also any movement inside feels as though all the organs in the lower region are moving and feeling very uncomfortable. I have a discharge but yet when we have intercourse, I sometimes need a lubricating jelly. I feel very small around the opening and my husband says it feels as though he is rubbing a bone along the top. He also agrees I feel tighter. My six-week check-up proved me okay but the hurting persists. I am beginning to feel that it's all in my head. I was in the hospital for an infection in the lower region, but they never knew exactly where. Please help me. I am desperate, not to mention my husband.

Comment—When a woman continues to have painful intercourse even though she has had medical advice, she should go back again and insist that she is still having a problem. By repeated visits perhaps the problem can be identified. The development of painful intercourse after pregnancy in a woman who experienced no difficulty before strongly suggests a medical rather than psychological cause. This would include the possibility of the painful scar caused from cutting the outlet to let the baby's head through the vaginal opening, or a tear in one of the ligaments which helps to support the womb. Sometimes in repairing the incision in the vagina to let the baby's head out, the tissues are tightened excessively which can cause some problem initially, but the vaginal outlet usually adjusts to this problem relatively soon, permitting normal sexual intercourse again.

Infections or inflammations in the bladder or vagina can, of course, contribute to painful intercourse. There is also a possibility that this woman is experiencing spasm of the muscles at the outlet of the vagina. A pelvic examination, however, should reveal this condition. In some women the muscles at the outlet of the vagina actually go into contractions at the time penetration is attempted. It would also

188

respond this way if a finger is inserted or if a doctor starts to insert a vaginal speculum to examine the woman. For this reason, the condition usually should be detected by an experienced gynecologist. When both the husband and wife appreciate what the problem is, by approaching sex carefully and not forcing the penis into the vagina, in the course of time the vaginal outlet will begin to relax to accept the erect organ and normal sexual relations can be resumed. Occasionally psychiatric counseling will be necessary.

Dear Dr. Lamb—I am a newlywed six months and now I should be quite used to making love since we are always doing it—meaning every day. The problem is really strange. We can make love once with no trouble and a second or third time it is like a sponge blocking the entrance of his penis. It feels like pins sticking me and becomes quite painful to the point of tears. We enjoy sex together and this is becoming a problem. Also, I am constantly getting infection after infection. We have both been checked but still they occur constantly. Is there any advice you could give me? We really need something done.

Comment—This girl may be experiencing the problem of honeymoon cystitis which I discussed earlier. The sensation of blockage of the entrance of the penis into the vagina strongly suggests that there is some degree of spasm at the outlet of the vagina. It's not likely that a physical barrier such as an unruptured hymen would be causing the problem or the difficulty would present itself with the first episode of sexual coupling.

The frequent intercourse that is common at the onset of marriage often irritates the urethra and causes cystitis (see Honeymoon cystitis). In the woman who has not had a baby, the thrusting of the penis bumps against the under surface of the bladder and sometimes irritates it. It could well be that this sets up a pain pattern which in turn causes spasm of the vaginal muscles. Recurrent infections in individuals who are highly active sexually is commonly observed. The infection is

189

in the bladder, and is called cystitis. It is not venereal disease, and it is not one of the vaginal infections that are common in women particularly after their early twenties.

Dear Dr. Lamb—Could you please answer this question for me? My boyfriend and I are planning to get married in the next few months, but we have had sexual relations. The question is what causes so much pain? I am very worried. I hope it is not my fault, but could you please tell me what causes the pain when first having intercourse.

Comment—The resolution to this problem is a good medical examination. Some young girls, even though they are engaging in sexual intercourse, have remnants of the hymen membrane still attached to the hymen ring. These can be inflammed or irritated and therefore painful during sexual intercourse. There are several other causes for pain during intercourse, but to identify them would require a competent medical examination. Previous sexual activity is not an excuse for avoiding a premarital examination and premarital counseling. Premarital evaluation should be carried out at least six weeks before the marriage to allow adequate time to correct any physical problems such as an excessively small vagina and a tight hymen. These measures will go a long way toward preventing painful intercourse which, if not prevented, can cause a lifetime of sexual maladjustment and often a marriage failure.

X

Male Anatomy Problems

THERE ARE NUMEROUS ANATOMICAL FACTORS which affect
men insofar as their sex life is concerned. These include
questions about the foreskin of the penis, undescended testicles, and questions related to circumcision; and a number of
letters indicate the constant concern of men about the size
of their penis.

PENIS SIZE

Dear Dr. Lamb—I have a son who is twenty-three, very
handsome, and the girls seem wild about him. He is
supposed to be married next month. The thing that
bothers me is his physical condition. He is healthy, but
his sex organs never developed more than an inch or
two. Do you think he will be able to hold a wife? My
wife tells me not to worry because his future bride
knows what she is getting, since she caught them in the
act and it was a natural act.

Comment—Men are about as concerned about the size of
their genitals as women are about the size of their breasts. In
both instances, these are visible evidences of the individual's
sexuality. There is a prevalent misconception among men
that a real "stud" is "well hung." The size of the penis is
equated with sexual capacity. The simple truth is it takes a
lot more to be a man or an effective lover than a large penis.

191

The size of the flaccid penis is relatively unrelated to its size in the erect state. In measurements done by Masters and Johnson the small penis tends to enlarge proportionately more during erection than the large flaccid penis. Thus the erect organs are more nearly comparable and there is not so much variation in size of the erect penis as might be suspected.

With the removal of sexual taboos and a climate that would permit finding out actual data, many myths concerning penis size disappeared. In his book, *Atlas of Human Sex Anatomy,* Dr. Robert L. Dickinson discusses this point and reports the result of measurements of the angle of dangle of the rigid digit and its length in 1,500 American white males. The average length of the erected penis is six and one fourth inches, and in 90 percent of the sample measured, the length was between five and seven and one half inches. The diameter varied between one and one fourth to one and one half inches. This means that 10 percent of the male population fell outside of these limits. Considering the normal statistical distribution of most samples, this means that about 5 percent of the men had erect penises that were shorter than five inches, and indeed, some considerably shorter have been reported.

There are two reasons why individuals are concerned about the size of their penises. During childhood the boy sees his father's sex organs. Since everything is relative to children, everything they see in childhood is larger than it is during adult life. The image of the large penis with the child's scope of measurement is implanted in the brain, and he always remembers his father as having an exceptionally large organ. The rest of his life he subconsciously tries to "measure up" to "the old man" and never quite reaches his childhood image of the size of his father's organ.

A second important factor is the misinformation about the areas of sexual response in the woman. The distribution of nerves over the skin and genital region that are most sensitive are limited to the outlet of the vagina and surrounding genitalia and about the outer one third of the vaginal vault.

This means that an erect penis that is only three inches long is capable of reaching most of the areas in the woman that are most sensitive sexually. Some women report that they like to feel the head of the penis thrusting against the cervix, but in general this is not necessary to achieve sexual stimulation of the female.

The truth is, the cervix is relatively insensitive. Physicians frequently snip out a piece of the cervix to examine the tissue under a microscope without any form of anesthetic and the woman is hardly aware that this is occurring. Such an insensitive portion of the anatomy is not likely to gain much from being bumped gently with the end of a long penis. Much of a woman's sexual response is also related to the foreplay, which involves the lovemaking, petting, fondling, and other activities which precede actual thrusting. Very often a woman judges whether her husband is a satisfactory lover or not on the basis of whether he has been able to stimulate her adequately prior to thrusting so that she is at the level of sexual response to achieve a climax.

If more men understood that the length of the penis during erection isn't so important, it would improve their sexual confidence and performance. Parents often worry needlessly about the size of their son's organ and they often make misjudgments on the basis of its size in the flaccid state.

There is another aspect of this problem: the question of the man with a very large penis. There are some of these. As far as diameter or circumference is concerned, with patience and time, most women can accommodate to a relatively large penis, even though it may not provide any more sexual stimulation. After all, the vagina is capable of delivering the head of a baby, so it's not likely to be severely challenged by the size of any man's penis as long as time is taken to allow the vagina to gradually accommodate it. This may take a number of sessions at the beginning of the sexual activity between a woman with a relatively small vagina and a man with a relatively large penis, but time usually solves this problem. The very long penis can limit, of course, the depth of thrusting that a man might be able to do. For example, reports of occasional men with an erect penis as long as fourteen inches suggests that in a woman with a vaginal vault of only seven inches, the penis is going to be considerably longer than is necessary to do the job.

In the man the greatest amount of sensitivity of the penis is at the head and the underneath surface of the shaft. Stimulation of the terminal six to seven inches is adequate for normal sexual responses.

Dear Dr. Lamb—My son is eight years old and is quite heavy for his age and weighs 100 pounds. His penis is of an exceptionally small size. I am afraid as he gets older he will be very self-conscious. Is there anything that could be done for this problem, like giving him hormones? I am afraid if this isn't corrected, he will get a psychological complex as he gets older. Would you please say something about this?

Comment—Parents start looking at their children early in life for signs of maturity. There seems to be a general misconception that to be early or first is best. This might be true if you are running a 100-yard dash, but it has very little to do with sexual development. If a boy is truly markedly overweight and has very small genitals, it's probably a good idea to have a medical examination. Fat little boys with small genitals sometimes have hormone problems. Laboratory tests can be carried out to see if this is the problem. Obesity is not beneficial medically at any age, and the parents of a fat little boy should seriously consider taking measures to eliminate his obesity early in life.

Many boys simply have delayed development. These are ones who are small in stature and generally small in all their bodily characteristics. They may also have a delay in the onset of sexual maturity. In American boys the onset of sexual maturity usually begins about twelve years of age, when pubic hair is usually first noticed. Shortly after this the other recognizable changes of puberty begin, including changes in voice, body size, and genital size. However, the onset of these changes is much later in some boys and may be de-

194

layed to nearly fifteen years of age, even though the eventual outcome is complete and normal development.

Certainly if mere delay in growth and generalized development is the primary concern, it is too early for any detailed evaluation until after age fifteen, and many doctors feel that starting puberty at age seventeen is entirely normal for boys. This, however, is about the outer limit before assuming that some problem needing attention exists.

Much is often made about the psycho-social aspects of delayed maturation in boys, but a lot of this is related to the parents' desire for their child to be "first." After all, their boy can't be very successful in the football or athletic arena if he is small, and this upsets dad usually more than it does the child. Other unenlightened parents begin to worry immediately about their son's sexual orientation. Parents can be informed of the facts but still respond emotionally. However parents might rejoice in late development, because studies have indicated that boys who mature later usually turn out to have greater personality flexibility and in many ways are psychologically more mature in later years than the "early bloomers." Apparently the "late bloomers" develop more internal resources in the process. Thus the early bloomer may be first but he may not be best.

Dear Dr. Lamb—I am a nineteen-year-old young man and happy in all aspects except one. To be very crude, my sex organs have not grown since I was very small. It was very embarrassing in gym class in school when I had to hide my body or be laughed at. They just seem to have stopped growing. I am too embarrassed to visit a doctor so I am writing to you. Could you please tell me what I can do about this problem, for example, shots, pills, or anything?

Comment—This is not an infrequent letter. A young man of nineteen is old enough for sexual maturation to have at least been well underway if not accomplished. An individual in this age group who has failed to mature sexually should see his physician whether he is embarrassed or not. Young men in this category often have a hormone problem. Not infrequently it's associated with a deficient amount of hormones from the pituitary gland, or master gland, which lies underneath the brain. In any case the correct diagnosis can only be made by a competent examination. Once the diagnosis is made, effective treatment can usually be initiated.

THE BENT PENIS

Dear Dr. Lamb—If I were you, I might consider that this letter came from some kind of crank or nut. I can assure you that such is not the case. It is a real situation and I am seriously seeking the answer. I am sixty-three years old and believe I have a normal sex life for my age. For several months, when I awaken in the morning with an erection, I have noticed that my penis bends upward in the middle at about a 90-degree angle. This of course is rare because I do not awaken with an erection very often. It does not interfere with sexual intercourse, because I seldom achieve a full erection during intercourse. I have not had any kind of injury that would cause such a phenomenon so I am considerably disturbed as to what could have caused it. Is it some kind of disease? Have you ever heard of such a case before? Is there anything I should do about it? There is no pain, no discharge, it just looks as if it has been broken.

Comment—I receive a number of letters about this problem. It occurs more often in middle-aged and older men, although it is known in young men too. Some normal young men have a penis which is curved downward, but does not bow or hook to a degree to interfere with sexual activity. This man describes a condition in which the penis bends upward, sometimes bending either to the left or right in a curved fashion.

This problem is called Peyronie's disease. The exact cause of the condition is not known, but it occurs when cordlike structures almost like scar tissue form in the center of the shaft of the penis, usually on the top side. These cordlike

196

structures cannot expand or stretch appreciably. When an erection occurs and the rest of the penis expands, then it has to curve upward. You can demonstrate the same principle by putting a piece of tape on one side of a long balloon. As the balloon is inflated, the tape cannot expand and the balloon curves upward toward the side where the tape is attached. The amount of curving and the location of the curve depend upon the length and location of the cordlike structures.

This problem is not related to cancer, venereal disease, or any other known disorder, but many people who write to ask about this problem are concerned about these possibilities. Very little is known about the treatment of this disorder. Fortunately, in some instances it will gradually go away. The angulation and rigidity of the penis can make intercourse difficult. Entrance of the penis into the vagina may be impossible, or if it is inserted it can cause considerable pain for the woman.

Some urologists have reported that doses of Vitamin E produce favorable results. It is difficult to judge these reports since in many individuals with this problem, the condition disappears spontaneously, whether or not medicine is given. The doses of vitamin E recommended for this problem are certainly not harmful, so it's worth a try. The usual method of treatment is to give 100 mg. (100 to 150 units) of Vitamin E three times a day.

CIRCUMCISION

Dear Dr. Lamb—I am a pregnant woman. My problem is that if the baby is a boy, my husband and my doctor both want to circumcise him.

My mother says this is a practice foisted upon American doctors by the Jewish instructors at medical schools, and that a man needs the foreskin for slack during sex. Furthermore, a man will lose most of his sensitivity and he needs the protection. She says we should have a partial circumcision if we have one at all and not to let a Jewish doctor do it because they take more off.

My husband says she is an anti-Semitic bigot, and none of her reasons are valid. He is circumcised and is a very good lover but I have no way of knowing how much better he would have been if he had not had this Jewish mutilation. Since this has come up he refuses to have sex or undress in front of me. My husband is deeply hurt and now feels bitter toward me and has a complex about circumcision. He claims many doctors and other experts say that circumcised men are better lovers.

Comment—Circumcision, or cutting away the foreskin of the penis, did not originate with the Jews. It was practiced by the ancient Egyptians and among Indian tribes in Mexico and South America, as well as the Australian aborigines.

Although techniques vary, a common procedure in newborns is to use a bell-like device which is slipped over the head of the penis; the foreskin is then drawn up over the outside of the bell. A ringlike device is slipped down over the bell and screwed down with pressure. This literally squeezes off the foreskin, which is relatively insensitive. The foreskin can then just be pulled away and the bell removed. This type of circumcision is called a clamp circumcision and does not cause the loss of a single drop of blood. There are variations in procedure including cutting away the foreskin around the bell. In older individuals the procedure is, of course, different and usually involves surgically removing the piece of skin.

Whether a man is a good lover or not usually is unrelated to the presence or absence of the foreskin. Men who retain their foreskin have just as much sexual enjoyment as men who do not have one. The factors that influence sexual activity are far more complex than merely the presence or absence of a little bit of skin. During the sex act, even in a man who is not circumcised, the foreskin normally retracts back of the head of the erected penis. There really isn't much to the thought that a man needs this extra skin for slack. In the course of having had multiple erections even early in sexual development, the skin will have stretched adequately to meet any requirements of this nature. The head of the penis remains sensitive in a circumcised male, as any man who's had this procedure would readily tell you.

The principal advantage of having a circumcision is cleanliness, which in itself is an adjunct to sexual activity. A natural substance, smegma, is formed around the head of the penis and can be trapped behind the rim in the uncircumcised male. It forms rather rapidly. Even so, with attention to hygiene on a daily basis, the uncircumcised male can keep himself relatively clean.

Considering the mechanisms of the female sexual response, it is inconceivable that it really makes any difference to a woman during the sex act whether or not her husband has been circumcised.

Although it is exceptionally rare, occasionally men develop cancer of the penis. This occurs more often in uncircumcised men. A tight foreskin can lead to problems in retraction of the skin and create difficulties both in hygiene and sexual performance. Sometimes if the tight foreskin is drawn back behind the head of the penis which then becomes erected, it can actually constrict the head of the penis and cause difficulties. This problem can be solved by doing a modified operation called the dorsal slit. This consists of cutting from the edge of the foreskin in a straight line back to the rim of the head of the penis. By making this one simple cut the diameter of the foreskin is markedly increased.

Dear Dr. Lamb—I am forty years old and have never been married. I have never been circumcised, and I am wondering if it is necessary before intercourse. Will it have any effect in preventing my wife from getting pregnant? I am planning to get married in four months and we do want children. I don't particularly want to be circumcised unless it is necessary.

Comment—Presence or absence of circumcision will have nothing to do with a man's capacity to cause his wife to get pregnant. Any man who is forty years old knows whether or not he produces semen. All that's required for pregnancy is for semen to escape into the vagina with sufficient viable

199

sperm at the right time to fertilize the ovum.

Dear Dr. Lamb—Is it possible for a man of fifty to be circumcised with little or no complications? He has trouble urinating and the skin has tightened up on the end of the penis and will not stretch properly.

Comment—A decrease in elasticity of the foreskin as the years progress is not an infrequent complaint in uncircumcised males. Keeping the foreskin lubricated to prevent drying of the skin and stretched offers some help. A man with this problem could have a dorsal slit operation which I mentioned in an earlier discussion. Certainly if the foreskin is so tight that a man is having difficulty urinating, such a simple surgical procedure is strongly indicated. This difficulty also suggests that the foreskin does not retract normally during sexual activity, and that there is undoubtedly a problem in maintaining adequate cleanliness.

UNDESCENDED TESTICLES

Dear Dr. Lamb—I would like information on a condition I believe is called cryptorchidism, when the testicles in the male fail to descend into the scrotum. Our son, aged twenty, has only one testicle, and we are wondering if he has another one or not. If so, can it be pulled down into the proper place in the scrotum? Will he be able to have children with only one testicle? He feels very guilty about having only one as he feels it has damaged his male ego and he is unable to have relations with any woman because of this condition. Please tell me what you think should be done.

Comment—During the early development period of the fetus the testicles remain inside the abdomen, and then usually at birth descend through the canal in the lower wall of the abdomen and into the scrotum. Occasionally one or both of the testicles fail to descend. If there is only one testicle in the scrotum, there is a good probability that there is another one either in the canal or within the abdominal cavity. The proper approach to this problem depends on the individual case. Sometimes the undescended testicle is removed entirely. In other instances, it is surgically placed into the scrotum. In young boys, in some instances, hormone therapy is used to bring the testicles down. Usually this is attempted before puberty to enhance the probability that the testicles will function normally.

If the testicles are brought down into the scrotum early enough, in many instances they will be normal. It is certain, however, that if they are left in the abdominal cavity long enough to produce male hormone, they will not produce normal sperm cells, and the man will be sterile. However, this does not mean that he will be unable to engage in normal sexual activity. It only means that the semen fluid will not contain normal sperm for pregnancy.

One testicle is quite sufficient in most instances to enable a man to father children. Not infrequently, if only one testicle remains in the scrotum, it will increase moderately in size to take over the function of both testicles.

Men often feel very threatened if there is anything unusual about their sex organs. Having only one visible testicle has its effect, particularly if the man doesn't understand that his one testicle is quite sufficient to provide the normal amount of masculinity and capacity to father children. There are two alternatives to this type of problem. The man can benefit from professional counseling and education along the lines I just mentioned; the other route is plastic surgery. I once knew a young pilot who had only one testicle. To solve his problem he had a plastic ball inserted in the scrotum so he would have two like everyone else. Sometimes plastic surgery of this type is the most rapid and effective means of psychotherapy and deserves the name "instant psychotherapy."

VARICOCELE

Dear Dr. Lamb—I am twenty-two years old and have a varicocele on the left side. It has been bothering me lately, not only physically but mentally. I haven't consulted a doctor yet, but I would like to get it removed. Is it a serious operation?

Comment—This young man is complaining about dilated veins in the cord to the testicle. They are analogous to varicose veins in the legs. A large varicocele can cause congestion of the testicle with resulting pain and aching. It can also cause sterility. The normal artery-vein relationship to the testicle functions to cool the blood and keep the temperature of the testicles lower than the temperature inside the body. The testicles are placed in the scrotum outside the body to keep them at a lower temperature so they will be able to produce normal sperm cells. If the temperature regulation of the testicles is interfered with, it can contribute to, or cause sterility. Obviously not every man who has dilated veins in the cord to his testicle, however, is sterile. It depends on the severity of the problem. If an operation is needed, it is relatively simple and effective.

Dear Dr. Lamb—I am experiencing cramplike pains in the area of my testicles. These are severe pains and last only a few seconds and occur with no regularity or pattern. Could this be prostate gland trouble? I am twenty-five-years old and have an office job where I sit almost all day long. Could this constant sitting have anything to do with the pain in the area?

Comment—There are many reasons for pain in the testicles, including the varicocele problem I just described.

One cause goes under the lay term "stonies," which refers to the congestion of the testicles that happens if a man is sexually aroused without orgasm. A young man of twenty-five years of age normally has a strong sexual drive and unless he has a means of sexual expression, this can contribute to the problem.

There are other causes for pain in the testicles including referred pain from conditions in the abdomen; for example, the passing of a kidney stone. Pain in the testicles does not mean prostate trouble.

202

INFLAMMATION OF THE TESTICLES

Dear Dr. Lamb—Could you give me some information on epididymitis. I want to know if you can get it from being under great stress. Do nerves or tension contribute to it? If you have it on one side, do you usually get it on the other? Can it be caused by frequency of intercourse, and does the condition of the blood have anything to do with the rate of recovery? How long does it last and what is the treatment for it?

Comment—Epididymitis means inflammation of the epididymis, the cordlike structure along the round body of the testicle. Like any inflammation, it can be caused by many factors, most usually germs. The infection is usually treated by giving an appropriate antibiotic.

Epididymitis is not caused by nervousness or the frequency of sexual intercourse. In fact, it has no relationship to sexual intercourse at all.

If the body of the testicle is also affected, it is called orchitis. Mumps can cause this condition. In all of these cases the treatment is totally dependent upon the cause. If it's orchitis with mumps, for example, antibiotics afford no relief and the principal treatment is giving symptomatic support until the illness subsides. If it is an identified bacteria that is causing the inflammation, then antibiotics are very useful.

SWELLINGS AND LUMPS

Dear Dr. Lamb—Two years ago I had a hernia develop on the left side. I had it operated on and immediately after the operation, my left testicle swelled and did not go down. As time went on, it continued to enlarge to the point where I had to go to another doctor. He said it was a hydrocele, which would only go down with surgery. A year after the hernia operation, I had it operated on and less than a year later it was swelling again. Could the doctor who operated on my hernia have done something wrong to have caused this?

203

Comment—Hydroceles, hernias, and spermatoceles are sometimes confused with each other. The hernia in the groin is caused by a loop of bowel that slips into the canal in the lower abdomen for the cord of the testicle. The bowel loop then can slip down into the scrotum causing apparent enlargement of one testicle.

A hydrocele is a sac of water which develops around the testicle. There are normally sacs of tissue there anyway, and sometimes they accumulate fluid. They can be drained by puncture to draw out the fluid or operated on with surgical excision of the sac.

A spermatocele is a cystlike structure filled with sperm cells that accumulates at the side of the testicle. The hydrocele can usually be identified by seating the patient in a dark room and placing a flashlight underneath the scrotum and seeing that the light shines through or illuminates the hydrocele sac as a red color. If it's a hernia the illumination from the flashlight will not be transmitted through the scrotum.

What probably happened in this man's case is that he had a hernia which the first surgeon repaired. Later, not because the surgeon did something wrong, but because of the nature of the structures in that area, he developed a hydrocele which may have been incompletely repaired with the second operation.

Hydroceles, spermatoceles and hernias are not cancer. Nevertheless any man who develops an enlargement or nodule on his testicle should immediately seek medical consultation rather than trying to guess what it is. In some individuals the enlargement of the testicle may be more important medically and require immediate attention, which may be life-saving.

XI

Breasts

THE CHANGING ATTITUDES about sex and human behavior are well illustrated by the changing attitudes about breasts. Prior to World War II, the limited availability of refrigeration led most mothers to breast-feed their infants. It was a common sight to see a woman sitting unself-consciously in a public place nursing her baby. The exposure of the mother's breast for public view was socially acceptable. It was less acceptable for women to smoke cigarettes, and a young girl who smoked cigarettes in public could be an object of community gossip. In the relatively short time that has passed since then, women now hide their breasts, would never think of nursing their babies in public, and yet a large portion of them smoke cigarettes, which is now considered to be socially accepted behavior.

The breasts are sexual organs in both men and women. The female breast develops under the influence of female hormones and the male breast can also be developed if the man is given sufficient amounts of female hormone. The breast in both sexes contains erectile tissue and stimulating the nipple will cause it to become erect. Clearly the breasts are something more than large specialized sweat glands. Stimulation of the breasts causes release of hormones in the body that in turn stimulate the uterus to contraction which may have a role in helping to milk the sperm cells up the uterus and into the tubes to initiate pregnancy. Thus the instinct to stimulate the breasts during sexual foreplay serves a basic physiological mechanism in inducing pregnancy. Breasts are also a source of many problems for women, including abscesses, discharges, sore nipples, tumors, and even cancer.

BREAST SIZE

Anyone who has received large volumes of mail from people concerning their medical problems will be aware that perhaps one of the most frequent concerns of women is the size of their breasts. Sometimes it appears that all women either think their breasts are too small, too large, or unequal. This preoccupation with the characteristics of the breast is normal. The breasts are one of the major physical signs of a woman's femininity. Like other important physical features, if a woman thinks there is something wrong with her breasts, it will affect her ego and self-image.

A large number of women overemphasize the importance men attach to breasts. While it is true that shapely breasts are an attractive endowment to a woman in the eyes of a man, most men are attracted to women because of their total personality and physical features rather than whether or not they have big breasts. A woman's concern about her breasts is a frequent motivation for cosmetic surgery. In addition to this relatively drastic approach to the problem, there are any number of padded brassieres and support structures commonly employed plus a lot of poor advice and downright quackery aimed at the woman who is unduly concerned about her breasts.

Dear Dr. Lamb—My breasts have always been very small. I have matured everywhere but there. I recently became married and for some reason I have become so conscious of my breasts being so small. My husband has never said anything, but I just don't feel like a woman. To me, I don't look feminine so I don't feel that way. I always turn out the lights before undressing because I am so ashamed.

206

The question I have to ask is is there any type of medicine or shot to take to enlarge breasts? I have tried bust exercises but while this does firm them, there is little difference and I did all the exercises every day just like the book and exercise course said. The reason I thought there might be is I've seen old movies of women on TV and they were small-breasted. Then you see them in movies now and they are large.

Comment—This woman's reaction is a typical response of a small-breasted woman who feels unfeminine. It points out well the identification that exists between breast size and femininity. No small number of women undress in the dark because they don't want their husbands to observe their small breasts. Frankly, most women are better off to accept themselves as they are. There is a lot more to being feminine and being a good wife than having big breasts. The size of the breasts has very little to do with the woman's enjoyment of sex in bed, or indeed her husband's pleasure. While stimulating the breasts during sexual activity is pleasurable, the simple truth is that the main event of the sex act doesn't require bosoms.

Exercises are of limited value, as are the various cream preparations. The only safe surgical procedure to increase the size of the breasts involves transplanting fat tissue from other parts of the body to the breast area. Usually fat is taken from the buttocks for this purpose. A plastic surgeon who does cosmetic surgery would be the right type of physician for this procedure. The names of plastic surgeons who do cosmetic surgery in a community can be obtained from the county medical society. Much of the breast is fat tissue anyway and all this operation really does is transplant some of the patient's own fat to the breast area. Problems of rejection do not occur with breast transplants of this sort because the tissue is the individual's own tissue.

Dear Dr. Lamb—My daughter is flat-breasted and she is very concerned about her condition. She is considering having her breasts injected with silicone, and I am afraid this could be harmful. Would you please tell us the dangers of silicone injections?

Comment—There are plenty of dangers. The U.S. Food and Drug Administration has reported four deaths from this procedure. The silicone material which is injected doesn't necessarily stay where it's placed and may enter the bloodstream and lodge in the lungs. It may also reach the brain. In other instances injections have caused massive abscesses which have subsequently required surgical removal of the breasts. The American Medical Association has taken a stand against silicone injections because of the complications they can cause. I receive many letters from women asking about silicone injections. At this writing, reputable physicians do not recommend them.

Dear Dr. Lamb—Could you comment on silicone implants to improve the bust. Are there any dangers? Whom could one contact for this treatment?

Comment—The silicone implants or other plastic or foreign material can be used to build up the breasts. This, however, requires a surgical procedure. Most plastic surgeons who do breast work prefer to use natural fat tissue from the patient for this purpose. This prevents a lot of complications and problems in some cases. I do not recommend silicone implants or other plastic materials for this purpose.

Dear Dr. Lamb—I am sure this question is of general interest to a lot of women. I asked my gynecologist about it and he just scoffed at me and said to be thankful I was healthy. My problem is I've gotten a bust increase plan and I'm not sure it's safe to use. I am 5'2" and 110 pounds, 32-27-36. Healthy but thin, and my chest is practically flat. Of course, I want bigger breasts but safely if possible. I don't want "large" breasts, but just enough.

I understand about creams, hormone injections, etc., and don't want to take anything. However, this plan is a series of exercises. Are exercises harmful to the breasts? A part of their plan is hydrotherapy to tone the breasts. You bathe the breasts in hot water, then alternate with a cold compress about twenty times before retiring. Is it wise to do this? They also claim irregular functioning of the adrenal and thyroid glands can have an adverse effect on the bust size. In my yearly checkup, wouldn't my gynecologist know if I had this problem? Please help me. Surely you can understand how horribly embarrassing this is for a woman to talk to a doctor in person about.

Comment—Contrast baths may help to tone up the breasts to a minimal degree, but they're not going to cause any significant increase in size. There is an endless list of different procedural recommendations advocated for increasing the size of the breasts. Most of them are complete phonies, and are in many ways comparable to the endless list available to men to increase their potency. When you start reading things of this sort, get hold of your pocketbook and close it tight. The contrast bath for the breasts is not likely to hurt them unless the water is too hot.

Dear Dr. Lamb—I am sixteen years old and as physically mature as I'll ever be. My problem is that I have practically no chest. I have heard that certain exercises can be done to increase your bust size. Could you please tell me some?

Comment—The exercises that do the most for the breasts really build up the chest muscles and improve the posture. Good posture does wonders for improving the bustline. It doesn't really improve the size of the bust, it just presents it better. Exercises that straighten the back and hold the shoulders erect help. In other words, if a woman holds her chest out, her breasts will stick out. To strengthen muscles to hold the shoulders back, she can do exercises which rotate the arms. This can be done by swinging the arms forward and upward, back and down, around and around. Another exercise is to hold the arms out straight and then forcibly contract the muscles between the shoulder blades, pulling the arms backward. Light stretch springs that athletes and weight training individuals sometimes use are helpful in building up the strength of the muscles between the shoulder blades. Learning proper posture habits, both for sitting, standing and walking, are important.

To strengthen the muscles on the front of the chest underneath the breast, put the palms of the hands together in front of the chest as if praying. Then push the hands against each other.

Dear Dr. Lamb—I wonder if you could help me. I lost a lot of weight, and since then my breasts have become very small. Is there anything I can do to enlarge them?

Comment—I include this letter as an example of the frequent complaint from women about weight loss. It is true that weight loss very often affects the breasts first. After all, a large portion of the breast is fat. The converse is not true. Making an effort to gain lots of weight will not necessarily increase the size of the breasts. All it will do is end up making the woman fat and less attractive.

Dear Dr. Lamb—I know you've probably had questions on this subject so much it bores you. It's the flat-chested woman problem, but I have heard and read that several groups of women have been given hormones over a period of time and their breasts have enlarged with no side effects. I would like your opinion on this subject.

Comment—The development of the breasts depends upon a number of complex hormone interactions. There has to be the right amount of hormones from the pituitary gland, from the thyroid, the adrenal, and the ovaries. Any hormone disturbance can affect the development of the breasts. I hasten to add, however, that the vast majority of women with small breasts have completely normal endocrine systems. In the normal female, giving her additional hormones is not likely to significantly affect her breasts unless they are given in amounts that are not normally recommended for health reasons. Women who have sometimes been benefited by hor-

210

mone administration are women who do have hormone imbalance. If a hormonal imbalance exists, it is proper to treat it anyway, irrespective of the size of the breasts. Some creams used for enlargement of the breasts advertise benefits on the basis of hormones. Creams containing female hormones should not be used unless they are given by prescription from a reputable physician. Most often if a woman really has a hormonal problem, the doctor will prescribe hormone pills or shots rather than a cream for breast development. To determine whether a woman needs hormone replacement requires laboratory study.

Dear Dr. Lamb—A woman wants larger breasts for many reasons. For one thing, her clothes fit better and you have a feeling of growing up. It gives you confidence to have larger breasts. For thirty-five years I was plagued with the problem of small breasts. I am a married woman and have given birth to seven children. While I was pregnant, my breasts went from a 32 to a 38. After birth, my bust was practically flat so I figured since my breasts became enlarged while pregnant, a woman must gain more weight and therefore the breasts would enlarge, but this is not true either. I tried exercise and nothing improved my bustline. Then I started to take "the pill" because I didn't want any more children. Lo and behold, my breasts enlarged to 38 again. Well, after taking the pill for two years, my doctor took me off the pill and my breasts shrank to nothing.

Comment—It is true that birth control pills will sometimes help to increase a woman's bust size. This is particularly true in older women when the ovaries begin to fail, and menopause is imminent. With the change of life, the breasts begin to decrease in size, starting to go back to the stage they were in before puberty. The birth control pills work because they contain female hormones that are normally produced by the ovaries. They delay the menopause and provide substitution therapy for the flagging ovary. Estrogen, which is a component of the birth control pills, also causes the body to retain salt and therefore fluid. This also contributes to an increase in the size of the breasts. Hormone replacement therapy of any type for women in the menopausal phase will help to maintain breast size.

Dear Dr. Lamb—I am writing concerning my fourteen-year-old daughter. She is developing very rapidly in her bust, more so than a girl of twenty-one years of age. She is small-boned and her body is small except for her breasts. I am very concerned because she is very self-conscious to the point where she is hunched over to hide them.

Is there anything that can be done medically to stop the growth of her breasts? I am very worried about her, especially where boys are concerned. She will not wear a swimsuit or go to the local pool at all. She is too young to have such a problem. What will it be like by the time she is fifteen years of age? She is already having a problem as far as the boys are concerned. I do not want to see her go through high school hunch-backed and self-conscious. Please help me. Any advice medically would be very much appreciated because I am sure there are other mothers with this problem.

Comment—And there are a lot of other mothers who would like to have part of this problem. Mothers are always concerned about their daughters' development. Girls who develop large breasts should be taught not to be ashamed of them.

There are no hormones or medicines that should be given to a girl to stop the growth of her breasts. That's the wrong approach medically. Women who have really tremendous breasts, and feel it necessary to do something about them, can have surgery once they have matured. The plastic surgeon removes part of the excess fat tissue and reshapes the breast. It is also necessary to relocate the nipple to maintain normal configuration. It is a reasonably complicated operation if a good and attractive result is to be produced.

212

Dear Dr. Lamb—I am fifteen years old and one breast is larger than the other. You can tell it. What's wrong and what should I do?

Comment—Usually the breasts aren't absolutely equal. It is said that the left breast is usually larger than the right, but from the number of letters I get from women who tell me their right breast is larger than the left, it's clear this isn't always the case. Unless the disproportion is really gross and distressing, the best thing to do is leave the situation alone. The only feasible approach would be to decrease the size of one or increase the size of the other by surgical transplant or surgical reduction. Breast size sometimes changes after pregnancy, also. Therefore, if a young girl has this problem she should hesitate about doing anything significant about it until after she has had her children. Then if she feels it is an important consideration, she should talk to a plastic surgeon about the problem.

Dear Dr. Lamb—I am fifteen and haven't worn a bra in almost a year. I'm not super well endowed but then I'm not super flat either. I've heard that going bra-less breaks down the cells and eventually causes one to get flabby. Is that true? I do bust exercises every night. Will that prevent flabbiness?

Comment—Once the breast has developed, going without a bra can indeed cause some difficulty. This is particularly true if the breasts are large or during pregnancy or during lactation. Dr. John Wulson of the University of Cincinnati College of Medicine commented on this in an article in the *Journal of the American Medical Association.* He states that the fibrous attachments in the breasts are stretched when they are left unsupported. Obviously, then, the heavier the breasts the more stretching and sagging will occur. Dr. Wulson states that the fibrous tissue does not retract to its former state regardless of how many exercises are done, and that the only way to prevent this drooping of the breasts from over-stretching of the fibrous connections is to support the breasts adequately with a suitable brassiere.

PAIN IN THE BREASTS

Dear Dr. Lamb—Please tell me is there any other disease of the breast besides cancer that can cause soreness in the breast of a woman?

Comment—There are many causes for pain in the breast and usually it is not cancer. Cancer develops initially in the breast without causing pain. A woman may experience pain in the breast which may be described as a tingling discomfort or prickling feeling about the time of puberty, before her periods, in the first few months of taking contraceptive pills, or in the early stage of pregnancy. It also occurs at the time of menopause, sometimes a number of years preceding it, without having any significance.

Dear Dr. Lamb—For about twelve years I have been getting a pain off and on in the side of my left breast. It only occurs for a couple of days periodically and not at the time my period would be due. Do you have any idea what may cause this discomfort?

Comment—There may be pain in the breasts from inflammation or lesser degrees of pain and discomfort for any of the causes I have listed in reference to the previous letter, but it should never be forgotten that the pain which is felt in the breast may be referred from some other source. There may be a sore muscle, a sore rib cage, or even pain from the heart which can cause pain in the breasts. More commonly, heart pain is in a more central location rather than at the side of the breasts, but when pain spreads over the entire chest it can also cause pain in the breast.

BREAST DISCHARGE

Dear Dr. Lamb—I have a breast condition that concerns me. The breasts discharge a fluid, one greenish and

214

one clear when they are compressed. I have been to several doctors and have had X-rays, Pap smears, and a breast culture. The doctors tell me not to worry but they do not explain the reason for the discharge. I am told it is difficult to treat and it will eventually go away. Could you explain what causes this and if it is cancer? How long will the condition last? I am thirty-three years old and have four children, and the condition has been present three years.

Comment—There are many things which cause a discharge from the breasts. This woman is describing a condition which is relatively common in women between forty and fifty-five years of age. The breast becomes lumpy and may discharge a greenish or blackish material. The lumpy feeling in the breast is not cancer. Technically, it is called fibroadenosis, or chronic mastitis. The condition can also cause pain and discomfort in the breast, especially preceding periods. Unfortunately, there isn't much that can be done in treatment, and the condition sometimes resolves itself. A well-fitting brassiere that provides adequate support is sometimes helpful.

Dear Dr. Lamb—Would you please comment on blood coming from the breasts. My breasts are very large and one of them has a discharge of blood. This has been going on for over a year, not all the time but once in a while. My doctor hasn't found any lumps or anything else. He also took X-rays which were negative and a biopsy which turned out to be negative. What could be the cause of the bleeding?

Comment—I have no way of knowing what this woman's bleeding is, but she did the right thing. Any evidence of blood from the breasts should cause a woman to go immediately to the doctor without delay for evaluation. It can sometimes be the signal of a cancer. In other instances, it is a small tumor growth in the breast which is not malignant, and the only way to diagnose it is through an immediate medical examination.

NIPPLES

Dear Dr. Lamb—I am a woman twenty-three with inverted nipples. Is this some kind of deformity? If not, is there any kind of treatment that can bring the nipples out?

Comment—When these occur in young women it is essentially harmless other than causing trouble in nursing the baby. The best treatment is to use the thumb and finger to draw the nipple out and do this daily for several weeks. A glass nipple shield can also be worn under a brassiere. If the nipple becomes retracted or puckered or twisted to the side in middle age or later, the woman should seek a medical examination because in this age group it may be indicative of a tumor of the breast.

CANCER OF THE BREAST

Cancer of the breast is the most common cause of death from cancer in females. In the United States one out of every fourteen female babies born is destined to get breast cancer, and one woman dies of breast cancer every twenty minutes. Because of the effectiveness of public education women are aware of the dangers of breast cancer and often frightened about this possibility. A number of controversies remain about the treatment of breast cancer, but one point stands out clear above all others—the earlier the diagnosis, the better the opportunity to correct the condition. This means that women should learn to examine their breasts for detection of lumps and that such examinations should be carried out regularly, preferably every month at a set time. A good time is about one week after the menstrual period. It also means women should have regular checkups by their physicians since women are not always adept at discovering lumps in the breast.

Some early signs of cancer cannot be detected by physical examination and for this reason, new methods are being developed. One is thermography which is based on the fact that a tumor area generates more heat which can be detected and

216

measured by specialized techniques. Other X-ray techniques include mammography and a technique which takes a special type of X-ray, processing it in a way not too dissimilar from the office copy machine to produce what is called a zeroradiograph. These additional methods may offer the opportunity to significantly improve the detection of breast cancer. Some enthusiasts have said it can boost the five-year cure rate from breast cancer by as much as 85 to 90 percent.

Lumps are not the only sign of cancer. Any woman who has a lump, a discharge whether it is blood-stained or not, a retraction or displacement of the nipple, a change in the character of the skin over the breast (often resembling an orange peel), or irritation around the nipple should immediately seek a medical examination. There are many other causes for a discharge from the breast, but it's best to let the physician do the examination and decide about its significance.

Dear Dr. Lamb—Please tell me what you can about breast cancer. Can it be treated in any way besides cutting into or removing the breast? That's out of the question, as far as I'm concerned. Would a doctor prescribe a pain killer if I choose to let the cancer go untreated?

I have two lumps. The first appeared about five months ago. They are the size of walnuts. One is a bit larger. I haven't been to a doctor, because I am afraid he would insist on cutting into the breasts. I suppose this all sounds terribly vain, but I would rather die than have my breasts removed. My husband wouldn't want to look at me, and I can understand that completely. I am not a youngster, I am forty-six and growing old, and dependency on others has not been my aim. I have lived a full life and my only child is grown. I would prefer to go with all parts intact and looking shapely if I can make my choice. I have no pain now, of course, but I suppose there will be some later.

How long do people usually live if they let the

cancer go untreated? Would X-ray treatments be effective? Should I go to a doctor and tell him what I've told you or wait until I have discomfort? Would a doctor accept a patient who refuses the treatment or operation that he thinks is necessary?

Comment—The attitude of this woman is dangerously naive. All lumps are certainly not cancerous, and she owes herself a medical examination to determine if she is needlessly worrying. Should she have cancer, her wish to preserve the shape of her breasts by forgoing surgery is based on incomplete knowledge of what cancer does to the body. Advanced malignancy of the breasts is not a pretty sight, so a woman who has cancer of the breast doesn't really have a choice about being shapely or not.

Unless the lumps were clearly not related to a cancer, the examining doctor would want to remove them and have them looked at under a microscope. Once the entire tumor has been removed and if it is not malignant, a very conservative doctor might be willing to stop there. Other surgeons would remove the entire breast and still others would go the route of a radical mastectomy which includes not only removing the breast but the lymph glands in the armpit and usually some of the muscles over the chest and into the arm in order to remove any areas where cells from the cancer might have spread.

There remains at this time considerable controversy about how radical breast surgery must be. In the current opinion of the American Cancer Society, a radical mastectomy is indicated. Some surgeons, however, are content merely with removal of the breast and a very small number of surgeons are content with removing only the tumor from the breast. In any case the best opportunity a woman has for a cure is early detection and early treatment, whatever treatment method is used. Hopefully, some of the early diagnostic techniques that I've mentioned at the beginning of this discussion about breast cancer will enable surgeons to find all of these cancer areas early and remove them, thereby making it possible to minimize the surgery and still have good

218

cure rate, but it is far too early at this point in time to say that this will be possible.

Dear Dr. Lamb—Please publish the fact that an inverted nipple may be a foreteller of cancer. If only it had been listed among the signs to watch for. I had read the signs many times about a lump and soreness, but this thing appeared quietly and I thought it was nothing to bother the doctor with. When a lump was found several months later I immediately sought help.

Comment—This is an accurate observation, and any change in the nipple causing it to be inverted, twisted, or displaced is a good reason to have an immediate examination of the breasts.

Dear Dr. Lamb—I would like to know what the latest and best methods are when searching for a lump in the breast of a twenty-one-year-old girl. I don't want the breast removed. What is the record or cure without it? Did you ever hear of a method I saw on TV that showed them painting something over the breast and if it turned a certain color it was cancer?

Comment—First, about how long a person will last with cancer of the breast if nothing is done about it. This varies a great deal depending on how malignant the tumor itself is. Cures for breast cancer are rated as five-year cures, so you could expect that a death would occur in less than five years. In most instances, it is a good deal faster. A lump, however, is not necessarily a cancer. The technique that this lady noted on TV is thermography, the material that's painted over the skin changes color in relationship to the temperature in the breast associated with the presence of a tumor.

The best way for a woman to examine her breast is to lie down and place a pillow under her right shoulder. Then using the flat surfaces of the fingers of her left hand, she should examine her right breast thoroughly. She should cover all the area of the breast by pressing it against the chest cage and feeling all of the different parts of the breast.

After she has done this, she should change the pillow to her left shoulder and using her right hand, examine her left breast. If she does this regularly at a set time on a monthly basis, she will soon become adept at examining her breasts and because she is familiar with her breasts may find a lump more readily than her doctor would.

The method is not foolproof and I have had a number of women write to me and say that even though they have done their examinations, they were found to have a lump in their breast which proved to be cancer. This is ample reason for a woman to have regular checkups by her doctor and not rely totally on her own ability to detect lumps. Nevertheless, every woman should follow this procedure because it can save her life if she finds a cancer early.

Dear Dr. Lamb—I recently discovered a lump on my breast which I had examined immediately by the doctor. He said it was a cyst and that's all and it would likely go away by itself and I am wondering just how long I should wait for it to go away and what if it doesn't? Also, what exactly is a cyst and what causes them? Do they ever become malignant? Do they have to be removed surgically?

Comment—Cysts of the breasts are relatively common. They are like a water blister inside the breast. No one knows exactly what causes them. If they are very large, they are sometimes removed from the breast. More recently some doctors have been draining the cysts with a needle. Not infrequently the cysts remain for long periods of time, and if they are removed they will be replaced by other cysts. It's just one of the characteristics of the breasts. They do not become malignant, but, of course, the presence of breast cysts does not guarantee that a malignancy can't develop elsewhere within the breasts.

Dear Dr. Lamb—About twenty years ago I discovered some lumps in one of my breasts, but these lumps disappeared. I have been having some trouble lying on my

220

side and there seems to be some swelling under my arm. I went to the doctor and he said it was chronic cystic mastitis and that there was no need for surgery. He said this might bother me for the rest of my life, and if it got worse to come in for shots. I have had very little trouble since then, but at times the breast seems sore. Can mastitis develop into cancer? I have had no more lumps, and at that time, the doctor said there was no cancer.

Comment—Chronic cystic mastitis is also called fibroadenosis. It is a form of chronic inflammation with a lumpy breast. The exact cause is not known. It often occurs in women between forty and fifty-five years of age and it does not develop into cancer. However, cancer can develop elsewhere in the breast. So like all other women, this woman requires recurrent examination and should examine herself regularly.

Dear Dr. Lamb—My husband likes to fondle my breasts. Having read quite a bit about breast cancer, I am wondering if this mutually pleasant play could be harmful.

Comment—No, it's not harmful. There have even been studies done on pinching the breasts of mice to see if the mechanical injury would increase the incidence of breast cancer, and it didn't. So fondle away.

Dear Dr. Lamb—Does venereal disease cause lumps in the breasts, and will the lumps go away after treatment of the disease?

Comment—Venereal disease does not cause lumps in the breasts. It can cause a lot of other undesirable things, but this is not one of them.

MEN'S BREASTS

Some men have prominent breasts merely because they're fat. A man can develop a tumor or even cancer underneath

221

the breast, but this is relatively uncommon. If men are given excessive amounts of female hormones, which has been done in the treatment of heart disease, it can cause enlargement of the breasts. There are a fairly large number of letters from young boys concerned about their breasts.

Dear Dr. Lamb—I am a fifteen-year-old boy and I have a hard knot on each breast. They're sore when they get hit. Other guys have them but mine stick out half an inch. It's been this way a year. Boy, how embarrassing!

Comment—About one out of three boys develop swelling of the breasts at puberty. This is a reaction to the increased amounts of hormones being produced at this time. Tender nodules in the breast area are common. In most instances they will disappear in twelve to eighteen months, but if puberty takes longer, they may persist for a greater length of time. These kinds of knots, however, seldom exist past eighteen years of age.

Dear Dr. Lamb—I am a nineteen-year-old male and I seem to have soreness in my tits. They are sore whenever anything is pressed against them.

Comment—This isn't particularly unusual. The nipples are more prominent in some boys than others, and they are really composed of erectile tissue. The nipples will stand upright if they are stimulated by light stroking, or when the man is sexually stimulated. Clothing which rubs against them constantly can irritate the breasts. When it was a habit to wear suspenders, these were often in a location to rub against the nipples and cause irritation. The skin over the nipple area can be kept moist by applying some form of lubricant, for example, a small amount of plain Vaseline, and this decreases the effects of friction of the overlying clothing.

Dear Dr. Lamb—What causes a man's breasts to enlarge like a woman's after seventy years? They are sore like a boil. I have a touch of emphysema, hardening of the arteries in the brain, the heart, and my legs, but I am most concerned about these female breasts I have developed.

Comment—As men get older, with decreased function of the testicles (often related to the finding of fatty deposits or hardening of the arteries to the testicles), the amount of male and female hormone produced is reversed. With the decrease in the male hormone and increase in female hormones, a certain degree of feminization of older men occurs. This includes changes in the voice and the possibility of more prominent breasts.

XII

Menopause – Male and Female

THE CHARACTERISTICS OF MENOPAUSE in the female are very well defined, although they vary in degree from woman to woman. There is some disagreement about whether or not a menopause occurs in men, but many authorities feel that a comparable series of events does occur in some if not all men. In women, the menopause is caused by involution of the ovaries and their functions. When the ovaries stop, the amount of female hormone that is available markedly decreases. There may still be some female hormone formed by the adrenal glands that rest over the kidneys.

The ovaries don't just suddenly stop one day, but gradually sputter to a stop, causing irregular menses and other symptoms of the menopause. The reason some women have less difficulty than others, apparently, is related to the amount of female hormone produced by the adrenal cortex. When the ovaries quit functioning, the woman tends to start to revert to her prepuberal physical characteristics.

Usually in the male, the testicles do not stop functioning, although there may be a gradual decline over a period of years. The slow, gradual changes are not so clearly identified as are the more sudden onset of symptoms noted in the female.

One way a doctor can tell how much female hormone a woman is producing is by looking at a smear taken from the vagina. According to the color and characteristics of the

224

cells, the doctor can tell whether the woman is deficient in female hormones or not.

SYMPTOMS IN WOMEN

Dear Dr. Lamb—Is there any way to stop hot flashes other than taking hormone shots? Last fall I started having them and finally they got so bad I had seventeen flashes in one day, and needless to say I was a miserable woman by the time I got to the doctor's office. I took shots over a period of fourteen days and felt fine and the flashes stopped. Now they are starting in again and are occurring one after another. The last three nights I had so many I got up in the morning completely worn out and sick. I am forty-three years old and do not have a regular period. I'd appreciate some information on hot flashes and what to do about them.

Comment—Hot flashes are one of the first symptoms of menopause. They are very troublesome for some women and not particularly noticeable in other women. The hot flashes may be confined to the face and the neck, or they may involve the whole body. In some women they include a flushing of the skin and may cause sweating. They last a short time and then the wave of heat disappears.

No one knows exactly why hot flashes occur, but a plausible explanation can be derived from the close proximity of the pituitary gland underneath the brain to the little center in the brain that controls body temperature—the body thermostat. The pituitary gland is directly related to the functions of the ovary. It stimulates the ovary to action and when it starts to lag, this affects the pituitary's function. The thermostat near the pituitary gland has the ability to dilate arteries in the skin and initiate body mechanisms that are normally there to reduce body heat. The body's thermostat can be affected by emotions, hot, spicy foods, and a number of different bodily functions.

Regardless of what causes them, severe hot flashes are

225

most uncomfortable. They are commonly relieved by giving female hormone, or estrogen, either in shots or synthetic female hormone preparations, such as stilbestrol by mouth. These hormones make up the difference between what is being produced by the ovaries and what the body needs. Some gland specialists think that the female menopause should be regarded simply as a glandular deficiency and female hormones should be replaced in this instance just as thyroid hormones are given to a woman with a low functioning thyroid gland. Hot flashes may occur intermittently throughout the menopause which may last from six months to as long as five years.

Absent or scanty menstruation is the other clue to menopause. Really that's what the word means, a pause or cessation in menstruation.

Dear Dr. Lamb—Since I reached the menopause, I am growing a lot of facial hair. What can be done about this?

Comment—This is not uncommon and it's related to the disturbance in balance between male and female hormones in the body. All of us have both male and female hormones. It's the ratio of the two that determines our masculinity or femininity. At the time of the menopause, the male hormones are unopposed by the actions of the female hormones, and facial hair often grows more prominent. Female hormones sometimes help prevent this problem. Of course, excessive hair on the face can be removed by electrolysis, for a relatively permanent destruction of the hair follicle, or they can be pulled out repeatedly on a recurring basis.

Dear Dr. Lamb—I am forty-one years of age and I have seven children. My youngest is nine. I think I'm going through the menopause. I was told because I am young and have not missed a period that I can't be going through the menopause. Is this possible? I feel like I am cracking up and have the whole world to fight. I have depressions and also no pep. Do I need help or am I going through the change? Not one of my children can stand me. I must be awful in their eyes and my husband's. Is it possible a person can go through this change and never miss a period? If not, I sure need some help of some kind.

Comment—A woman's menstrual periods need not completely disappear for her to begin the menopause, and forty-one is certainly not too young for the menopause to occur. In rare cases it can begin in a woman's latter twenties.

Emotional instability is a frequent accompaniment of the menopause. This doesn't mean a woman is going to lose her mind or have serious difficulties, but she is often more irritable and depression is common. It is sometimes difficult to differentiate between the emotional symptoms that accompany the menopause and those indicative of a psychiatric problem. Tests like the one I mentioned, in which cells taken from a smear from the vagina, are studied, help to identify how much estrogen is being produced and are an aid in determining whether or not menopause is beginning.

Dear Dr. Lamb—I am forty-three years of age and in my menopause. Over the past two years I've gained considerable weight. I've tried several diets, exercise, and watching what I eat, but I can't seem to lose any weight. I menstruate regularly but each month I seem to flow less. Could this be because of my weight gain? I've heard of people gaining weight during the menopause. Is this possible? Is there any particular diet that I should follow to lose weight?

Comment—Weight gain is frequently part of the picture of the menopause. The body mechanisms slow down. The woman, at this period of her life, often has raised her children and has less need for physical activity. She is often frustrated and even bored with her decreasing responsibilities. Boredom and frustration stimulate eating. This, combined with even a minimal decrease in physical activity, gradually adds fat stores to the body. Because of the tendency of women to gain fat deposits during the menopause and there-

227

after, a woman is well advised to take particular pains to decrease her calorie intake during this stage of her life. She should avoid high calorie foods which, in the main, are those foods that include large amounts of fat and concentrated sweets like sugar. Too many calories of any kind will contribute to the obesity problem.

At the same time a woman is gaining weight, she will frequently have a decrease in the size of her breasts. It seems like all the fat goes to the wrong places. This is also a good time for a woman to improve her regular exercise program. She should start paying increased attention to exercises that improve her posture. This includes the same exercises that I mentioned earlier in helping to improve the posture to enhance the bustline. These exercises should be carried out to strengthen the muscles between the shoulders and in the back. Basically these are exercises that involve arching the back between the shoulder blades and strengthening the muscles between the shoulder blades. If these muscles are strong enough, they will help prevent the degeneration of the spine that is so common in Caucasian women and results in the buffalo hump that affects about one out of four American women by the time they are sixty years of age. It's very difficult to do very much about these problems once they have occurred, but a preventive program can help a great deal.

Dear Dr. Lamb—I am forty-six years of age and until about six months ago, my sexual desires were great, but now I think I am going through the menopause because I haven't had a menstrual period for several months now and my sexual desires have decreased more than half. Before, all I had to have happen to me was for my husband to kiss me, and I was ready for the bed. Now I don't get any feeling or desire. Do you think my menopause has something to do with my not desiring sex as I used to? Perhaps I can take some kind of vitamins to get back my nature. I sure miss my sexual relations. Do you think my sexual relations or desires

228

are over? I think I'm still young enough to enjoy sex.

Comment—Some women experience a decrease in sexual desire during the actual menopause. But once the menopause is over, many women experience a marked increase in sexual drive. This, however, is not always the case. Some women continue to have a decreased interest in sexual activity. In general, individuals who have enjoyed a satisfactory sex life before the menopause will continue to do so in later years, even though they may have a decrease in their sexual desires during the menopausal phase.

Dear Dr. Lamb—I am forty-four years old and went through the change about a year ago. I had no trouble at all, only hot flashes at times. My husband said that when a woman went through the change, her muscles relaxed and intercourse wasn't the same as before for him. Is this me or him?

Comment—It's true that a lot of women have relaxed muscles around the vaginal outlet about this time in life, but it is not because of the menopause. It's most often caused by pregnancies, particularly if multiple births have occurred. Incidentally, the overstretched muscles can be tightened by simple surgical techniques. It is true that if the vagina is too lax, it has limited ability to provide friction or contact sensation to the penis, and the man's enjoyment of sex will be significantly decreased.

Dear Dr. Lamb—I am fifty-three years old and have not menstruated for two years and have had hot flashes, so am going through the menopause. Is it common for a woman's breasts to ache off and on through the menopause and afterwards?

Comment—Yes, women do have tingling and aches in the breasts as long as five or ten years before the menopause. It seems that intermittent sensations of this sort are also seen before menstrual periods and in other circumstances, but the problem is more pronounced near the menopausal years. It disappears after the menopause.

Dear Dr. Lamb—I would like to know if there is any change in the uterus at or after the menopause besides the stopping of the menstrual flow.

Comment—Yes, the uterus decreases in size. In general there is a tendency toward complete involution of the female sexual apparatus. The uterus gets smaller, the cervix thins out and gets smaller, and unless vigorous sexual activity is maintained, the vaginal vault will shrink. The external lips of the vagina will shrink in size and the fat pads around the vagina will diminish. This is accompanied by changes in distribution of fat in the body, a loss of breast size, and an increase in hair on the face. It's a pretty complete involution. Many of these changes can be significantly delayed or even prevented in some degree by the continued administration of hormones.

Dear Dr. Lamb—I had a hysterectomy a little over a year ago and I was wondering since I have my ovaries and I am now forty-two years old, will I still go through the menopause? I get hot flashes and headaches a great deal and also some itching, and I feel depressed too. My doctor doesn't believe in hormone shots. Do you think I should see another doctor? He also says I am too young to be going through my menopause.

Comment—Yes, a woman who's had a hysterectomy with the ovaries still intact will continue to have normal sexual cycles without menstruation until she reaches the menopause. At that point she has the likelihood of experiencing the same symptoms that other women do during the menopause, including hot flashes and nervousness. As mentioned in commenting on previous letters, forty-two is certainly not too young for a woman to go through the menopause. Some doctors do not believe in hormone shots. I do.

HORMONE THERAPY

There are a number of unanswered questions about the administration of hormones to women during the menopause and in the post-menopausal period. There is a strong body of evidence that suggests that replacement of female hormones helps at least to delay or prevent part of the aging process in women. Some doctors refuse to give patients female hormones regardless of their symptoms, resorting merely to hand-holding and encouraging the women to "tough it out." No doubt if men had similar symptoms there would be a lot more hormone replacement prescribed and a little less hand-holding.

Dear Dr. Lamb—Recently I read a pamphlet about the effects of the menopause. The pamphlet described the menopause as a deficiency disease with serious consequences for the great majority of women. They listed serious problems brought about by the lack of female hormones, which included tissue weakness, excess cholesterol in the blood, degeneration of the bones, joint disease, diabetes, and high blood pressure. They stated that if a "maturation index" indicated a below normal estrogen level they advocated the woman should take female hormones which would result in periods with planned bleeding. Would you please give me your opinion on the importance of hormone replacement. Does it really help prevent endometrial cancer?

Comment—Not only will female hormones alleviate the symptoms of the menopause whether the menopause occurs naturally or as a result of surgery, it will help to prevent such problems as degeneration of the bones which is common in post-menopausal women. (I also recommend that women should drink at least a quart of fortified skim milk or its equivalent in calcium daily because a calcium deficiency increases the likelihood of having degeneration of the spine fourfold.)

Caucasian American women seem to be protected against high cholesterol levels and fatty deposits in the arteries during the childbearing years, but they are not protected after the menopause and by the age of sixty-five they have the same frequency of these difficulties as men do. However,

231

simple replacement of female hormone alone hasn't been demonstrated to reverse this problem in all women. The change seems to be somewhat more complex than that. Some authorities advocate giving small amounts of thyroid hormone at the same time female hormones are given because the thyroid gland also lags a bit at this point in life. Be that as it may, unless there is a real reason not to give it, I believe the weight of evidence is on the side of those who advocate replacement of female hormones at the time of the menopause and in the post-menopausal phase of life. It is not established that female hormones cause any type of cancer (see Cancer).

Dear Dr. Lamb—Will you please write something about older people taking hormones. Do you think it is harmful for them after sixty-five?

Comment—No, it is definitely not harmful. It can be very beneficial in some women. In the absence of sufficient female hormones, the vaginal vault dries out and makes continuation of an active sex life painful or impossible. This can also lead to changes in the vaginal vault secretions, causing the vagina to be susceptible to infections. When you consider the entire range of things that can occur because of a decreased amount of female hormones in the menopausal and the post-menopausal span of life, there are strong arguments for giving these hormones.

Dear Dr. Lamb—Today I went to my gynecologist for my checkup and it seems I am too old to take birth control pills but too young for estrogen pills because of a fluctuation in my hormones. So what in the world am I to do if I get crabby and tense and can't take anything for it?

Comment—Birth control pills act by substituting female hormones that are cyclically produced by the ovary during the menstrual cycle. In doing this they prevent the maturing of ova and thereby prevent pregnancy. Since they work because they are female hormones, it's clear that they can also help prevent the symptoms of menopause. Many doctors put their patients on birth control pills and leave them on them, thereby delaying the actual appearance of the menopause.

Many women on birth control pills don't even know whether they have reached the menopause or not, because they will continue to have a regular menstrual cycle with regular recurring menstrual periods at the time the birth control pills are stopped. Therefore, there really isn't such a thing as being too young for estrogen and too old for birth control pills.

Dear Dr. Lamb—What did you mean by saying in your column that hormones are two-edged swords? I am going through the menopause early (aged thirty-four) and have been having deep depressions and suicidal thoughts as was the lady that you wrote about in your column. However, my family doctor put me on hormones and it changed my world. Now I hear from friends that their doctor said he wouldn't let them take hormones because it might cause cancer. With your statement on it being a two-edged sword, I am a little uptight.

Comment—Hormones can be a two-edged sword in more ways than just the question of cancer. Estrogen causes the body to retain salt and therefore fluid. Some women object to the swelling which is associated with this process. Some doctors feel that giving female hormones increases the likelihood of developing cancer, but this question is far from settled. There is even some evidence that they may protect against cancer.

Dear Dr. Lamb—Because of a malignancy I have had breast surgery. Also, I have had a complete hysterectomy but there was no malignancy. I am in my early fifties and now I have a hormone deficiency and my husband's and my sex life has diminished to practically zero. On account of my breast surgery my doctor refuses to let me take estrogen which I feel would help.

I'd like your opinion on taking female hormones and what can be done to restore sexual activity.

Comment—It is common for doctors not to give female hormones to a woman who has already had breast cancer or uterine cancer. This has been a long-held view in medicine. Recently these views have been challenged, and it may well be that the balance of hormones in the body is more important than whether or not hormones are present. It could be that estrogen, in certain circumstances, even protects against breast cancer. Dr. John Burch and Benjamin Byra at Vanderbilt University School of Medicine carried out a study of over 500 women who were given estrogen preparations for nine years or more after they had had their ovaries removed surgically. While some of the women did develop breast cancer, it occurred almost a full decade later than it occurred in comparable women who were not using estrogen. The doctors' studies strongly suggested that there was an apparent delay in the onset of breast cancer in women who had received estrogen. It should be remembered that a large number of women will develop breast cancer anyway, and its occurrence in a woman who has been receiving estrogen does not mean it is caused by the estrogen therapy. The Vanderbilt study even suggests that it may protect women for a number of years against breast cancer.

In a similar study on lung cancer, Dr. Jack Chalon, Dolores Loew, and Louis Orkin at the Albert Einstein College of Medicine have amassed information that suggests estrogen may protect women from lung cancer. This may provide the explanation for why men smokers develop lung cancer more commonly than women smokers. In any case the entire concept that female hormones cause cancer is open for reconsideration.

MENOPAUSAL MENSES

Dear Dr. Lamb—I went to see a gynecologist and he scheduled me for a D&C. He didn't answer my questions, and I hate to undergo even minor surgery if it's not necessary. Is it normal for a woman of forty-five to spot and stain between periods? Is the cessation of periods a gradual thing? What is normal or average for a woman approaching the menopause?

Comment—This woman's doctor is doing the right thing. Mid-menstrual bleeding in a woman past forty should certainly be investigated. It is true that women can have mid-menstrual bleeding as a breakthrough phenomenon in their menstrual cycle. The midpoint is about the time ovulation occurs, and at this time there may be a significant decrease in female hormones temporarily causing the bleeding. However, nonmenstrual bleeding can also be caused by cancer or other problems. The proper approach is a diagnostic study such as the doctor is doing in this instance. At the menopause it is common for the periods to become irregular, sometimes scanty and sometimes profuse, or they may be missed intermittently.

Dear Dr. Lamb—My question is this, when can one become certain that the menstrual periods are finished? Some medical journals and doctors say between the ages of forty-five and fifty, but generally speaking, what do you say?

Comment—About 75 percent of American women have their menopause between the ages of forty-five and fifty. A few will have their menopause a little later, and a number considerably earlier. It is most unusual, however, for a woman to be menstruating past her middle fifties. It is very difficult to tell when a woman is really through having her periods, because she may not have any for quite a while and then suddenly have a period. This is because the ovarian function does not stop abruptly, but gradually sputters to a halt.

The difficulty in determining when a woman's menstrual period stops is exemplified by the following letter:

Dear Dr. Lamb—In a recent letter in your column you stated that a lady who was fifty-seven years old and was still menstruating was very unusual. This resulted in another lady sixty-two years of age writing in who claimed that she was still menstruating. In January I'll be seventy-one years old and have normal menstrual periods, though I may skip a month or two or more.

The first time I started menstruating again was in 1959, seven years after my menopause. I had a Pap test and a thorough examination which was completely negative. In 1966 I started spotting occasionally, but no excessive bleeding and the Pap test was negative. The spotting has a tendency to continue between periods, though I keep it fairly well under control with warm salt douches, advised by my family physician. It would be interesting, scientifically, under these circumstances, to know if the possibility of pregnancy exists. Too bad I've been a widow all these years. I am blessed with very good health and have never had a serious illness or surgery. I have the pep and energy comparable to a woman twenty years younger.

Comment—This certainly is a very unusual case history, and the fairly regular continuation of menstruation even though she is seventy-one years old strongly suggests that she still has functioning ovaries. There are a lot of women, of course, who continue to have menstrual periods because they are on birth control pills or sequential pills used to treat the menopause and post-menopausal phases of life. This woman's letter suggests that her periods are unrelated to taking medicines.

MENOPAUSE AND PREGNANCY

A common concern of women at the time of menopause is whether or not they can still get pregnant. Many of them, from their letters, would like to be able to enjoy sex without needing to take precautions against pregnancy.

Dear Dr. Lamb—I am a woman of forty-nine years and last year I had gone nine months without a period. After the nine months I had one. Now I have gone seven months without one. Please help me and tell me if I am still able to bear a child. How long does a menopause last? How can you tell if you cannot have any more children? I have heard that fifty-two is the limit. Someone told me that a woman's childbearing span is only thirty-five years and you can count from the year a woman begins her cycle up to her present age to tell if she can still get pregnant. I'm forty-nine and began menstruating when I was fourteen, so this would be thirty-five years.

Comment—In dealing with biological events, it is a good idea not to be overly positive. Nature has a way of fooling us. It is most unlikely for a woman past her middle fifties to get pregnant. It is also most unlikely for a woman to get pregnant if she's gone through the change of life and hasn't menstruated for two years. A seven-month period isn't a long enough test. It is not true that a woman's childbearing years cover a thirty-five-year span. In general, the woman who starts menstruating early continues to menstruate later, thereby giving her a longer childbearing span than the woman who begins menstruating later in life.

Dear Dr. Lamb—A group of women, all menopausal or post-menopausal and on estrogen of one type or another, have different opinions on the effects of estrogens. These are all fairly intelligent women with high school educations or more. Our ignorance is enormous. Since we are probably a good cross section of American women this lack of information must be amazing. Can you help educate us? One forty-five-year-old woman, seven years after a hysterectomy and on a hormone, claims a woman on hormones can get pregnant even after the change of life if she has gone through the natural change of life instead of surgical change.

Another woman three years after her last period just recently started on hormones and claims this is impossible after the menopause because the ovaries are no

237

longer producing eggs and no medication will ever cause a post-menopausal woman to be pregnant again.

Still another woman not on hormones of any type claims from a reliable source that a seventy-five-year-old woman became pregnant after taking estrogen and claims also that ovaries become functional again and will produce eggs when a woman is on estrogen. Would you please straighten us out?

Comment—It is not true that a woman who has completed the menopause and is then placed on female hormones can become pregnant. She is just as sterile as the woman who had a surgical menopause. It is difficult to tell when the menopause is actually over, but usually a woman who has gone through all the signs of menopause, falls within the proper age group, and has not menstruated for over two years is highly unlikely to ovulate or get pregnant. Thus the woman who said pregnancy was impossible after the menopause is essentially correct. It's true that once the menopause is completely over, the ovaries are no longer producing eggs. It is also true in this state that female hormones will not cause ovulation.

There is no reliable record of a woman seventy-five years of age having a child. The menopause is caused by the ovaries degenerating or aging. They stop producing eggs and female hormones. The two functions are directly related. Occasionally women get pregnant during the menopause simply because they didn't realize that they were not yet through the menopause; that is, the ovaries were still producing eggs occasionally. Another common mistake that women make is to assume that because they are not menstruating, they are not ovulating. No small number of women who are not menstruating have been surprised to find out all at once that they are pregnant.

Dear Dr. Lamb—I started taking birth control pills at age forty-one to regulate my menstrual periods. Is there any possibility of my becoming pregnant if I discontinue the pills?

238

Comment—Yes, there is a possibility that a woman in this age group going off birth control pills could get pregnant. A woman on the pill has a lot of difficulty knowing whether she has gone through the menopause or not. The birth control pills replace her hormones and she is having a pill-induced menstrual period regularly. A woman in this age group, if she really wants to stop taking the pill, should do so under her doctor's advice, but use other means of birth control while she is being studied to find out if she can get pregnant or not.

In the final analysis women who are concerned about this problem should have an examination by their doctor or gynecologist. By specialized tests, including looking at cells taken from the vagina, he can get a very good idea of how active her ovaries still are. Many doctors will still avoid giving a woman an absolute answer about whether or not she can get pregnant because, as I mentioned earlier, nature has a way of fooling us.

MALE MENOPAUSE

Dear Dr. Lamb—Would you please comment on how to cope with men going through the change of life. My husband is very depressed and not interested in anything, plus his sex life isn't what it used to be. He is fifty-three years old. Do you think hormones could help him?

Comment—Many doctors don't think that men have a menopause, while others do. Nevertheless in the middle years of life, many men experience a marked decrease in their sexual capacity. No small number of them in the American population have recurrent problems of impotence. Emotional problems come along at this time in life for many men. They realize that the goals they had set earlier in life cannot be obtained. The changing from the self-image of a vigorous young man to a man whose youth is spent can be a tremendous ego blow. An identity crisis can result, comparable to the identity crisis women have when they face similar changes.

The identity crisis associated with the middle and later years is not greatly different from that experienced in teenagers. In both instances there are drastic changes in the body and in the future roles the individuals play in society. Because of the numerous environmental factors involved, it is difficult to say whether a middle-aged man's depression is related to the change in life or not.

The only way to tell whether a man is truly having a change in life caused by changes in the body is by measuring the hormone levels. If there is a significant decrease in male hormone accompanied by an increase in the hormones formed by the pituitary that normally stimulate the testicles in the man or the ovaries in the woman, then he has a comparable hormone pattern to that noted in women going through the change in life. When these changes do occur in a middle-aged man they are usually caused by degenerative changes in the testicles. I would like to stress again that these degenerative changes in the American male population may be directly related to the decrease in blood supply caused by blockage in the arteries from fatty deposits. When a definite decrease in hormones is identified, hormone replacement is helpful.

Dear Dr. Lamb—What is the latest thinking on male hormones (testosterone) for a man seventy years old for poor circulation and male climacteric. The reason I am asking is that my personal physician gave it to me once a month or more frequently, and I felt fine. I entered a home for retired people and the doctor cut me down to once every six weeks and I have failed physically in spite of his saying that I'm in good shape. He is afraid I will develop cancer of the prostate gland. I have no prostate trouble at this time.

Comment—It is true that in older men with a decreased testosterone level, providing this hormone will improve their

240

vigor and vitality, not only in the sexual sphere but as far as the strength of their muscles is concerned and their general interest in life. There is always some concern about cancer of the prostate which occurs frequently enough as men get older, and it is true that male hormones stimulate the growth of the cancer once it occurs.

In the absence of any prostate difficulty, however, physicians would have different opinions about the advisability of using male hormones. Given in small doses to maintain physical vigor in the presence of a definite deficiency of male hormone, I would recommend them. They often markedly improve the sexual capacity and alleviate middle-aged depression. They are not indicated, however, in a man who has normal levels of testosterone and obvious normal hormone production. Men who have sexual dysfunction with normal hormones usually have other problems, often with a psychological basis.

XIII

Female Surgery

BECAUSE OF THE FREQUENCY of torn or relaxed muscles after childbirth, fibroid tumors, unexplained bleeding, and other problems, many women undergo surgery on their female organs. Many women are fearful about what these procedures do to their sex life and health.

STRETCHED PELVIC MUSCLES

As a woman grows older, particularly if she has had several children, the muscles which surround the vagina become stretched, and the ligaments and structures which hold the uterus in place may be torn or stretched, causing the "womb" to fall.

Dear Dr. Lamb—I am twenty-seven years old. I have been married for five years and have two children, aged four and three. For the last two and a half years my sex life with my husband has not been enjoyable. The reason is that I am too large for his penis which is not that small. Could you tell me of some cream I could use to make myself smaller? Is this condition strange? Can it be helped?

Comment—No, the condition is not strange. It's due to the stretching and tearing of the vaginal muscles during childbirth. The more relaxed the muscles and structures are, the

242

more difficulties will be encountered in enjoying sex. The weak muscles will not be able to provide sufficient contact or grip the penis.

At the time of childbirth many obstetricians will make an incision through the muscles at the outlet of the vagina to let the baby's head pass through without tearing any of the muscles in this area. After the child is born, the incision is sutured together, thereby preserving the strength and tone of the muscles. If this is not done, occasionally a woman will tear the muscles in this region as the head comes through the vulva. Such tears can be sutured in place but complications can arise if damage extends into structures that are difficult to repair.

Creams and lotions have no effect on this condition; the only effective remedy is a surgical repair. Technically, it is called a pelvic floor repair. If the uterus has "fallen down," it can be re-anchored in place and all of the structures in the pelvic region, including the bladder and rectum, can be placed back in their normal positions and the structures in that area reinforced. The success rate of this surgery is high, and most couples report a significantly improved sex life. Many doctors object to performing this operation, however, until a woman is through having children because the next pregnancy can undo everything they have done.

Dear Dr. Lamb—I have an unusual problem and I hesitate to go to a doctor because of the embarrassment of it. I tell myself that's silly but I still don't go. I am thirty-two and have had three children, and I've had this problem two or three years. The wall between the vagina and the rectum has weakened. I have trouble with elimination because the bowel movement seems to form a pocket that bulges into the vaginal area. The only way I can start elimination is to press with a finger on this pocket. Otherwise, on urgency, the pocket just grows larger. Obviously this causes problems during intercourse. Can I do exercises to strengthen this wall or will this require an operation?

243

Comment—This letter exemplifies another condition resulting from stretched structures and muscles in the genital area. The rectum is directly behind the vaginal vault. When these muscles have been overstretched through childbirth, the separating wall may protrude into the vaginal canal. The result is exactly as this woman describes. It might be considered as a hernia of the rectum into the vaginal vault. The sac-like pouch that protrudes into the vagina enlarges as fecal material builds up and is not normally eliminated. Pressing on the pouch is merely a mechanical way of reducing the hernia so that a bowel movement can occur. The proper treatment for this problem is surgical correction of the damaged structures in this area.

Dear Dr. Lamb—What is a prolapsed uterus and what causes it?

Comment—This is the condition in which the uterus has fallen down into the vaginal canal because of overstretching or tearing of the ligaments and supporting structures around it. It usually occurs in women who have experienced childbirth. In extreme cases it may prolapse so far that the cervix will be near the mouth of the vagina.

Dear Dr. Lamb—I am sure there must be lots of women who have the same problem I do. I am fifty-four years old and have a fallen bladder which protrudes out as large as an egg. It is pretty uncomfortable. Seven years ago I had an operation that did help some, but for the past two years it is even worse than it was before. Would you suggest another operation or is there anything that can be done without surgery?

Comment—The bladder is in front of the vaginal wall, and it can herniate into the vaginal vault through torn and stretched structures just as the rectum does from the other side of the vagina. Repair of the muscles and structures in this area eliminates the herniation of the bladder into the vaginal vault. The operation is a hernia repair.

The herniated bladder is commonly called a cystocele. The

244

portion of the bladder that extends into the hernia traps urine that can readily set up infection of the bladder or cystitis. All hernia-type operations are not always successful the first time (although there is a high success rate), and in some instances a second operation is needed.

Many readers are concerned about whether these problems are related to cancer—they are not. They are simple hernias related to torn and stretched muscle, ligament, and tendon structures. The problems they cause are the result of the hernias and are mainly bladder infections, difficulty with sexual relationships, and problems with bowel movements.

Dear Dr. Lamb—I am a female who was almost pulled apart when our daughter was born and have had some problems since. After a lot of lifting, the problem is much worse and I almost lose everything. I am in my seventies and am fighting an operation. I wear a pessary most of the time and lose it often. What I'd like to know is if there are some kinds of exercises that would help correct this problem?

Comment—No, these torn structures cannot be corrected by exercise and they are not helped a great deal by a pessary. Think of this as the same problem as a hernia. You can't correct a hernia in the groin (inguinal hernia) by exercise. Heavy lifting in the presence of a hernia will aggravate the problem and it can aggravate the hernia of the structures into the vagina as well. The surgery really isn't dangerous. Depending on how much has to be done, it may take a little bit of time, and a woman who is in reasonably good health even though she is in her seventies could tolerate such a procedure very well.

It is difficult to retain a pessary if the hernia of these structures into the vagina is fairly marked. The pessary will simply be pushed out and rendered useless.

Dear Dr. Lamb—My husband has been dead several years and I have taken douches, but the douche part won't go in as far as in the past. It seems to strike the end about two thirds of the natural length as compared to the past. As I am getting married I would like to know what to do about it, because it isn't right. Will it work out all right or should I see a doctor?

Comment—Obviously, this woman should see a doctor.

It is likely that one of the structures in this area has herniated into the vaginal vault. She may be striking the cervix if the uterus has dropped down, but certainly if she has a hernia of the type that produces obstruction to the nozzle for douching, she cannot expect to have satisfactory sexual relations until the problem is corrected. She may get some benefit out of sexual relationships when she is lying on her back, particularly if the pelvis is elevated because the herniated structures will tend to fall back into place in this position. It sounds like she needs surgical repair of a vaginal hernia.

The three basic vaginal hernias, then, are herniation of the cervix, uterus or womb into the vaginal vault from above, herniation of the rectum into the vaginal vault from behind (rectocele), and herniation of the bladder into the vaginal wall from in front (cystocele).

SURGERY AND VIRGINITY

Dear Dr. Lamb—When an unmarried woman has a hysterectomy, complete or subtotal, is she considered a virgin or does this surgery take her virginity away from her?

Comment—I am absolutely astonished at how many women are so concerned about the appearance of virginity that they even fear surgery because of the possibility that they might lose their hymen. There are several ways of doing a hysterectomy and whether or not the hymen would be destroyed in the process depends upon the approach used. If the cervix is left in place, the hysterectomy may be carried out through an abdominal incision. This would mean the vaginal vault would not need to be entered, and an intact hymen, if one is there, would be undisturbed. None of the structures in the vaginal vault would even need to be touched with such a sur-

246

gical approach. If the cervix is taken out, again it depends on the approach which is used. Many gynecologists now prefer to take the cervix out with the rest of the uterus, thereby eliminating the future possibility of cervical cancer.

If a vaginal hysterectomy is done, the approach is through the vagina, and in that event, of course, the hymen would be removed, if one were present. If such a woman had never been examined or handled sexually, the vagina would be so small that a vaginal hysterectomy would be more difficult, if not impossible.

Dear Dr. Lamb—Can you tell me how an examination is performed on a twenty-year-old virgin to determine if she has cancer of the womb?

Comment—By virgin, I presume this reader means a woman with an intact hymen membrane. Quite obviously the membrane is going to be stretched enough to admit instruments into the vaginal vault for a complete examination, or else the hymen will actually have to be removed. If the hymen happens to be very loose and stretchable (which it is in some women even if they have been sexually inactive), theoretically the hymen can be stretched and the instruments slide under its edge.

If the doctor is going to be able to look at the cervix, near the top of the vaginal vault, he is going to have to look into the full length of the vagina. To dilate the uterus and curette out material from the lining of the uterus (dilatation and curettage, commonly called D&C), he is going to have to introduce instruments through the cervix. Even a new procedure which essentially washes cells out of the cavity of the uterus would still require an insertion through the cervix.

As far as the companion question which I receive frequently on this—after such a procedure is a woman still a virgin—it seems to me that the definition of a virgin constitutes something more than whether or not the hymen membrane is intact. There are many ways that the hymen can be torn, including athletic activity, which have nothing to do with the sexual habits of the person. If one's definition of a

247

virgin is one who has not had sexual intercourse, then diagnostic and surgical procedures have nothing to do with the question of virginity.

Dear Dr. Lamb—Is it possible for a woman of thirty-nine to still find fulfillment of her sex life after a complete hysterectomy? What about a partial one?

Comment—This is a very frequent question. Many women either do not understand what the hysterectomy operation does or else they do not understand their sexual organs and what is used during the sex act. A partial hysterectomy removes the body of the uterus; a complete hysterectomy takes out the cervic portion as well as the body of the uterus. If only the body of the uterus is taken out, the cervical stump stays in place and there is no real need for the vaginal vault or any of its structures to be disturbed. If the cervix is also taken out, the end of the vaginal vault where the cervix is normally located is sewed shut. This leaves a normal, full-length vaginal barrel.

The operation does not in any way affect the muscles of the vagina, the external lips or vulva, the clitoris or any other part of the female anatomy. The lubrication for the sex act comes from the wall of the vaginal vault, so the normal moisture will remain. The sensitivity for response to the sex act is mediated to the brain and the rest of the body through nerve fibers that are located in the outer one third of the vaginal vault and the external genitals, far away from where the surgery is done. In short, there is absolutely no reason why a woman who has had a hysterectomy can't continue to have a completely satisfying sex life.

Some women who have had this operation have an improved sex life because they no longer need to worry about getting pregnant. Also, there will no longer be any menstruation since menstruation is the shedding of the lining of the uterus. As long as the ovaries are left in place, the normal female cycle and production of hormones will occur, including ovulation. There simply will be no place for the eggs, or ova, to go.

248

With the ovaries in place the woman will in time go through menopause, unless hormone replacement is provided. This is often done in other women who have had no surgery at all. In short, if only the uterus is removed, with or without the cervix, a woman will still have her normal sex drive and maintain the capacity to have an orgasm or multiple orgasms without fear of pregnancy.

Dear Dr. Lamb—I had a hysterectomy due to adhesions. The doctor left in the right ovary. Will I go through the menopause change or will I have some kind of physical or mental change? I am thirty-five years old.

Comment—If both ovaries are removed during a hysterectomy, it is more than a hysterectomy and in this instance a woman will have a surgical menopause unless she receives hormone substitution. As long as one ovary is left in place and is still functioning normally, the menopause will not be precipitated by surgery. When she reaches the time for decrease and gradual cessation of her ovaries' functions, then she will go through a menopause like other women.

Dear Dr. Lamb—A little over a year ago I had a hysterectomy. Since then I am sure that I see a difference in the size of my breasts. Is this possible?

Comment—The breasts change size in women for a variety of reasons, including the simple loss of body fat. As a woman gets older and enters the menopause, the bust usually decreases in size. Simple removal of the uterus alone should have no effect on the size of the breasts.

Dear Dr. Lamb—I have had a partial hysterectomy and I still have my ovaries and tubes. Is it possible I could get pregnant in the tubes? I have heard of such pregnancies.

Comment—It's possible, but not very likely. The fertilization of the egg by the sperm occurs in the tube. Thus, if surgery is carried out immediately after the egg has been fertilized and before it has entered the uterus, the pregnancy can develop

249

in the tube. The impregnated egg literally has no place to go. The possibility of having a tubal pregnancy, then, is relatively slight and involves only a short span of time, since the egg can only last about six or eight hours and the sperm only lasts about forty-eight hours. If a woman has not had intercourse for at least three or four days before surgery, it would seem impossible for her to develop a tubal pregnancy.

Dear Dr. Lamb—A little over two years ago I had a rectocele repaired. The surgery was a complete success with one exception—relations with my husband since then have been painful. I dread the ordeal from one time to the next. Sometimes I am almost tempted to tell him I can't keep having relations with him, but I know that is not the answer. Is there anything—anything at all, surgically or otherwise, that can help in this situation? We had such a good sex life before I had the surgery and I am so hopeful that there is something that can remedy this situation.

Comment—A few women have painful intercourse after surgery, and it is not always psychological. It can be caused by painful scars or in other instances it can be because of mechanical difficulties that follow in the wake of the reconstruction program. To really identify the cause one needs to know exactly where the pain is located and what aggravates it the most. This needs to be combined with a very careful gynecological examination. This is a mechanical problem that can often be corrected. It is worth going back to the doctor about and going back again and again if necessary until the problem is resolved.

I have received some letters from individuals who tell me that their doctors have said they will continue to have pain with intercourse the rest of their lives. I don't agree with this and feel that if a doctor does not make a genuine effort to determine the cause of painful intercourse that occurs after surgery, particularly in a woman who had previously enjoyed a normal sex life, the woman should probably seek a consultation with another physician, preferably a competent gynecologist. If there is no medical reason for the problem, then professional counseling by a psychiatrist is indicated.

ENDOMETRIOSIS

Dear Dr. Lamb—I am in my middle forties and recently underwent surgery made necessary by a retroverted uterus and ovaries diseased by endometriosis. My daughter is in her middle twenties and has been having the same kind of symptoms I had at that age. She has been to a gynecologist who tells her there isn't much he can do but give her something to ease her pain and discomfort. This is what I was told twenty years ago. Is there no treatment for this malady?

Comment—Endometriosis affects a lot of women. It's really an aberration of nature. The specialized tissue which lines the uterus is called the endometrium. It is this specialized tissue that enlarges and prepares for the pregnancy and sloughs off during menstruation. Women with endometriosis have some of this same specialized tissue located in other places in the body besides the lining of the uterus. The specialized tissue can be in the tubes or ovaries, or even in other parts of the body. It swells and enlarges at the same time the lining of the uterus enlarges during the menstrual cycle, and it decreases in size and sloughs off and undergoes changes at the time of the menstrual period. When it is located in a sensitive area, like one of the tubes, it can cause pressure and pain during its swelling phase. If it increases in amount it can actually destroy the structure that it's located in; for example, the ovaries.

When endometrial tissue is located in the ovaries, it often causes pain and even interferes with ovarian function. The tissue in the tubes can cause blockage and create problems with pregnancies. Unless the displaced endometrial tissue is located where it causes real trouble, the doctor may elect to leave it alone. After the menopause the endometrial tissue subsides, and it is no longer activated. In other instances, depending on the location and severity of the problem, the

251

doctor may feel it is necessary to remove the displaced endometrial tissue.

CANCERS AND TUMORS

The female organs are a major source of cancer in women. The most common location for cancer in women is the breasts, and the second most common the cervix and uterus. There are also lumps and tumors that are not cancers which develop in the uterus.

Dear Dr. Lamb—I have had two fibroid tumors in my uterus for four years. Each day they seem to bother me more because they are growing. I think they bother me mentally because I know I have them. I have been to doctors and they don't seem too concerned, as if there isn't anything to worry about unless they cause some serious change. I would like to know just how serious they are, or can be. Should they be removed immediately after discovery? An answer may help me, physically and mentally.

Comment—Fibroid tumors are fairly common. A tumor means a mass or lump. A tumor composed of fibrous tissue (much like the type of tissue you find in scar tissue) is called a fibroid tumor. They commonly develop in the uterus. They can develop during pregnancy without necessarily preventing a normal birth.

Fibroid tumors are not cancerous, and we use the medical term, benign, to indicate this. Since they are not malignant, doctors don't become very excited about them unless their presence in the uterus causes difficulty. Even a small fibroid tumor in the uterus can cause excessive bleeding, and when this occurs, sometimes it is necessary to remove the tumor. Depending on the woman's age and other factors, including how many children she has had, some doctors will remove the uterus. If a tumor is very large and located in the right position, it can produce pressure symptoms on the bladder, causing frequency of urination. Or it can cause a heavy pres-

252

sure feeling in the lower abdomen just by virtue of its size and weight. If it's a small one without symptoms in an older woman, the doctor may elect just to leave the tumor alone. I am sure there are many women who suffer needless anxiety about fibroids, not realizing that a true fibroid tumor is not a malignancy.

Incidentally, some women ask if a fibroid tumor will interfere with intercourse. The answer is no. The tumor is in the uterus. Intercourse uses the vagina and is unaffected by the uterus unless it is prolapsed or herniated into the vaginal vault.

Dear Dr. Lamb—Recently I had a Pap test as part of my routine female examination. The report came back suspicious. I have had a conization of the cervix with the report being carcinoma in situ. Could you please explain what conization of the cervix is and what carcinoma in situ means? I was told this will be repeated after my baby is born. Can this affect my child in any way? How often will this be repeated in the future? I am twenty-nine years old.

Comment—This lady's letter points up the value of the Pap test, which is a very simple procedure. Cells are scraped from the lining of the vagina or near the cervical area and examined under a microscope. From the characteristics of the cells the examiner can get some idea if there are any early signs of cancer, even though the physical examination may be entirely negative. Many cancers are detected early in this way, and this woman's story is one of those.

Carcinoma in situ means, literally, cancerous growth in its natural place that has not extended to other tissues. In other words, it is still a small, localized area confined only to that one spot.

Conization of the cervix is literally cutting out a cone of tissue. In this instance the cone is cut out in such a way to include the localized area where all the cancer is located. Without the Pap test, the cancer might not have been detected that early, and this simple procedure might not have been possible. The simple procedure described by this lady will not affect her baby. If the cancer had not been detected by the Pap test and had progressed rapidly, then more serious measures might have been necessary in the course of her pregnancy which could really have caused some problems.

Dear Dr. Lamb—Is it necessary for me to have a Pap test yearly? My doctors say that women over forty should have one, but does this apply to all women regardless of whether they have been married or have had any sexual relations. Since getting a sample is a painful ordeal, for me at least, and I am fifty years old and unmarried, is it really necessary?

Comment—Cervical cancer is more common in women during their active sexual years. It is less common in nuns, for example, than in married women in the same age group. There are still so many unknowns about the causes of cancer that it is difficult to say whether this is meaningful or not. Women who do not have intercourse, however, do develop cancer even if it is at a lower rate. Because the testing procedure really isn't that difficult compared to the problems that can be created from failure to obtain an early diagnosis, it seems to me all mature women should have a regular checkup. During the checkup, an opportunity is also afforded for checking the breasts which are the most common site of cancer in women.

Dear Dr. Lamb—I am very thankful to you for the advice in your column suggesting all women who have problems with a bloody show to see their doctors at once. I had a complete examination and the test was okay. A month later I had a bloody show, and after reading your column, I went to my doctor. He performed a D&C and found a malignant tumor. I was treated with radium and later by a complete hysterectomy. Thanks to your advice, as my doctor said if I had waited six months it would have been too late, I am now fully recovered and am very thankful.

Comment—This letter illustrates dramatically how important it is for a woman to go to a doctor for a checkup if she has unexplained bleeding. This is true even if she has had a recent examination within the past few weeks. Early diagnosis of a malignancy does save lives, and early diagnoses can only be obtained by seeing the doctor when any sign develops which suggests the possibility of cancer.

Dear Dr. Lamb—I am fifty-nine years old and had a complete hysterectomy. The doctor I have been going to for the past four years for checkups says I do not need a Pap test since I have had a complete hysterectomy, so he doesn't give me one. Is this true? I hope so because I hate those Pap tests.

Comment—There is room for some difference of opinion since it still is possible for a woman to develop a cancer of the vagina. However, these are relatively rare. The common cancers of a woman's genital tract are of the uterus and cervix. If a hysterectomy has removed both, which is usually called a complete or a total hysterectomy, the main source of cancer is eliminated. A woman should have a regular checkup, however, so that at this time she can have a breast examination as well.

Dear Dr. Lamb—Much has been written on cancer of the cervix, but little has been written about cancer of the endometrium. How soon after symptoms appear does this tend to metastasize and to what organs?

Comment—It is true that cancer of the cervix has been well publicized, and this is responsible for a dramatic improvement in curing women with this problem. The number of deaths from endometrial cancer is about the same as the number of deaths from cervical cancer. However, as recently as 1940, there were eight cancer deaths from cervical cancer to every one death from endometrial cancer. This dramatic change in ratio is a direct result of the education of the public to obtain early examination.

Cancer of the lining of the uterus, or endometrial cancer,

255

is silent unless it starts bleeding or is already metastasized with cancer cells in other parts of the body. This is one reason why at the first sign of bleeding a woman should go for an examination. In the past the only way a doctor could examine the inside of the uterus was to do a dilatation and curettage (D&C). This meant dilating the cervical opening, the mouth of the uterus, and scraping out tissue which could then be examined under a microscope. This requires hospitalization and a general anesthetic because it is a painful procedure.

A new development promises to change all that. A doctor now can study the cells inside the uterus as a result of an office examination. It will probably do for cancer of the endometrium what the Pap test did for cancer of the cervix. The test was developed by Dr. L. Clark Gravelee of Birmingham, Alabama. Gynecologists are enthusiastic about the test because it can be done in the office. It uses a modified syringe. The tip is slipped into the uterus and, through a jet washing suction-type device, removes cells from the lining of the womb which can then be studied. This is a fairly rapid procedure.

To provide some idea of the woman who should have such tests, one gynecologist described the high-risk candidates for endometrial cancer as women with any of the following characteristics: over forty, post-menopausal, menstruating after forty-five, obese, diabetic, hypertensive, childless, and women on long-term estrogen therapy. Nearly 800,000 women in the United States will eventually develop endometrial cancer. This method holds promise of significantly reducing the hazards of this type of cancer.

XIV

The Prostate Gland

EVERY MAN WHO LIVES LONG enough develops a firsthand acquaintance with his prostate gland. It can be acutely infected, causing severe pain, fever, prostration, and sexual difficulties. It can be chronically inflamed and cause trouble continuously over a period of years. It can enlarge to a point that it shuts off the urine flow, and finally it is a frequent location of cancer in men. Despite all these negative factors, it does serve a useful function. It secretes large amounts of fluid that transport sperm cells during orgasm. The substances in the prostatic fluid provide nutrient for the sperm cells as well. The rest of the seminal fluid comes from the seminal vesicles, two little storage pouches directly adjacent to the prostate gland. More recent studies also indicate that the prostate gland forms substances which protect the male from urinary tract infections. This may be one explanation why men are less prone to urinary tract infections than women.

Before puberty the prostate gland is relatively small, not much bigger than the end of the little finger. With the bodily changes brought on by puberty the prostate gland enlarges under the influence of a male hormone. It grows until it reaches about the size of a walnut. It is located at the outlet of the bladder and is wrapped around the urethral tube that comes out of the bladder through the penis to drain urine. It is this location that enables it to cause trouble when it begins

257

to enlarge. As the prostate gland closes down on the urethral tube, it literally squeezes off or acts like a clamp around the urethral tube to prevent draining the bladder. The prostate gland itself is somewhat like a sponge, composed of crypts for the storage of prostatic fluid. These crypts are really glandular structures that drain through multiple openings in the crypts into the urethral tube. At the time of orgasm the prostate gland contracts and, like squeezing a sponge, the prostatic fluid is squeezed into the urethra for ejaculation.

The tubes from the testicles come up with the cord from the testicles underneath the skin in the lower part of the abdomen, enter the canal into the abdomen, and go directly to the prostate gland. The right and left tubes terminate on each side of the prostate gland, draining the sperm cells directly into the prostate. In this way the sperm cells are literally washed into the crypts with the prostatic fluid for ejaculation. Just before the tubes reach the prostate, they connect with the drainage tubes from two small saddlebag-shaped structures lying on each side of the prostate gland. These are the seminal vesicles, which also provide fluid that is ejected into the terminal part of the tubes in the testicles and literally flush out the last part of the sperm cells into the prostate for the last part of the ejaculation.

SYMPTOMS OF PROSTATE TROUBLE

There are several different kinds of prostate difficulty. Acute inflammation of the prostate is common in young men. It causes pain between the legs just in front of the rectum and can cause pain in the lower part of the abdomen. Because it is an acute infection, it may cause generalized symptoms of illness including fever, sweating, and weakness. Frequently pain or burning on urination occurs. Sometimes at the end of urination there will be a drop of blood or pus. These acute infections are caused by germs such as those normally present in the bowel.

Because the prostate gland is located just underneath the bladder, it can be felt through the wall that separates it from

258

the rectum. The finger is inserted into the rectum and can be moved freely around the margins of the prostate gland to determine its size and hardness. During acute prostatic infection, the gland may be enlarged and tender to examination. Ideally, a specimen of prostatic fluid is obtained by massaging the prostate through the rectum. This material is then placed in a culture where the germs will grow and can be identified. Once a germ is identified, it can be treated with various antibiotics and medicines to see which ones are effective treatment. Then the medicine is administered and the acute infection is cured. At other times doctors use antibiotics or medicines that cover a wide spectrum of different germs. With proper treatment most of the acute types of infection can be cured rapidly, with no lingering effects.

However, some infections are chronic in nature and cause trouble over a long period of time. Also the prostate can be chronically irritated and congested without any germs being present. A common cause of this, particularly in young men, is sexual excitement without sexual release. During sexual excitement there is an increased blood flow to the pelvic region. The increased amount of blood in the area tends to cause tissue swelling or engorgement. With sexual release the blood flow to these areas is sharply curtailed, the excess blood is drained off, and the congestion disappears. Prolonged, repeated sexual excitement without release maintains congestion and causes the prostate to be slightly enlarged and soft. Nature has a remedy for this problem that doesn't require a trip to the doctor's office.

The common enlargement of the prostate gland is not an infection. It is simply an overgrowth of the gland which may or may not be associated with cancer cells.

Dear Dr. Lamb—Some four years ago at age thirty-four I suddenly developed what has been variously described as "recurrent or chronic prostatitis" or inflammation of the prostate. There is quite severe discomfort much of the time, and although I have been given several drugs and had regular massages and have taken hot baths daily, it continues with occasional severe flareups which are almost completely debilitating for several days. Sometimes my specimens are "full of pus and blood," yet the lab can't culture anything. Doctors say this isn't unusual, but it makes treatment difficult and I must "try to live with it" and eventually it will "burn itself out." Well, after four years I am extremely tired of living with this and strongly desire a cure. It's difficult for me to understand why in this day of modern medicine something can't be done to relieve me of this misery. Would you tell me if there are any new treatments which might be tried?

Comment—This is not an unusual story. Once the prostate gland has been infected for a period of time, it can develop a continuous low-grade inflammation. Treating this problem is aggravating to both the patient and the doctor. As I mentioned in the answer to the previous question, it is sometimes difficult to determine which antibiotic will prove effective against the infection. Prostate massage is commonly done for this problem, hoping to relieve the congestion and swelling by manually stimulating the prostate to contraction and expelling its fluid. Hot sitz baths are usually prescribed in the hope of relieving the aching and other symptoms. Basically, this problem is the male equivalent of the woman's problem of chronic mastitis.

Dear Dr. Lamb—I would like to know what causes blood in the urine. Would the prostate gland have anything to do with it?

Comment—Blood in the urine can be caused by many things. An acute prostate infection can cause a few drops of blood. However, blood in the urine always calls for an immediate medical examination without delay. The blood can come from the urethral tube if it's been irritated for any reason, from the bladder, or the kidney. In addition to being a symptom of prostate infection, it is also a manifestation of more serious diseases including tuberculosis of the kidney or cancer of the kidney. It is this latter possibility, in particular, that should cause anyone who has blood in the urine to visit his doctor for a complete medical examination within a few hours or days.

Dear Dr. Lamb—What would cause an intense burning pain when I urinate with a persistent, burning sensation afterwards, along with the feeling that I have to go again to no avail? I assure you there is no VD problem involved and I am fifty-seven years old, male, and a Christian. I am afraid that I need a prostate examination, but after friends told me about how much it hurt them, I am scared to go to the doctor. I would certainly appreciate your advice.

Comment—Burning on urination merely means that the acid content in the urine is irritating an area in the prostate or urethral tube that has been damaged or irritated in some way. It can be caused by prostate trouble which may simply be an acute infection. The only way to find out is by medical examination.

Examination of the prostate gland is not necessarily painful. A great deal can be learned about the prostate gland by simple rectal examination. A rectal should be part of the examination in all adults (male and female). Not only is this examination helpful in identifying prostate trouble, but it is also important in early detection of cancer of the rectum. This latter disorder occurs at any age, including young adults, and if detected promptly by this simple examination, can be cured.

A urinalysis is also indicated to determine if an infection is present. Depending upon these findings, the doctor might have to do other procedures which are, indeed, less comfortable. Even these are not as bad as allowing a potentially significant disorder to go uncorrected.

Dear Dr. Lamb—I am fifty-five years old. On my last physical examination my doctor told me my prostate was somewhat swollen, but nothing to worry about for a while. I have to get up twice every night and sometimes it takes me five minutes to urinate. During the day when I am working I have no trouble. What makes me have this trouble at night?

Comment—There are several disorders that cause a person to get up at night to urinate, including diabetes. This symptom alone doesn't necessarily mean a person has prostate trouble; however, it certainly is one of the signs. In addition to having to get up at night, a person may have to urinate frequently, even during the day.

The characteristic of the stream during urination helps to identify prostatic obstruction. The enlarged prostate obstructs the flow of urine to the point where urination proves difficult. It is often difficult to get the stream started, and the man will have to exert more effort. Once the stream is started it lacks the force of normal urination and is frequently difficult to shut off completely.

With progressive obstruction to the outflow of urine, the bladder retains more and more urine and fails to empty completely when a man urinates. Normally, urination involves the contraction of muscles in the bladder much like a squeeze bulb on a giant syringe. As the walls of the bladder contract, the urine is squeezed out through the penis. Because of the obstruction, the entire function of the bladder changes. The overstretched bladder has trouble contracting properly and doesn't exert enough force to completely empty itself. Because of this the person constantly feels like he has a full bladder, and returns frequently to the bathroom to try to relieve himself. The weak bladder muscles can squeeze out only a little each time. The condition progresses until sometimes men have enormous bladders by the time they seek medical attention. By passing a hollow tube, or catheter, through the urethral tube of the penis into the bladder drainage is established. An extra quart of urine in the bladder is not unusual, and in some instances a whole washbasin of urine can be drained out.

Prostate enlargement can affect only one side of the prostate in such a way that it doesn't squeeze down on the urethral tube. In this instance the man will not experience

262

any major difficulties in urination. Also, even though the prostate doesn't enlarge on its external surface, it can still be enlarging in its center, gradually squeezing down on the tube. Enlargement of the prostate is so common that one out of five men will have prostatic enlargement by the age of fifty, and four out of five by age eighty (this does not mean cancer of the prostate).

PROSTATE OPERATION

Dear Dr. Lamb—I would like to have some information on just what the terms "cystoscopy" and "transurethral resection of the prostate" mean in plain English. Also, if the prostate is operated on, what happens to the tubes from the testicles? If the prostate is removed, can it be replaced?

Comment—Cystoscopy is simply a procedure to look into the bladder. A little steel rod is passed through the urethral tube (through the penis in the male or directly through the urethral tube in the female) and into the bladder. The rod is designed with a light on the end of it so the doctor can look directly into the bladder. This way he can locate an area of irritation, a spot that's bleeding, or a tumor on the side of the bladder. He can also determine the characteristics of the lining of the urethral tube.

Transurethral resection is one of the ways of removing prostate tissue. It really means cutting away (sectioning) across the urethral tube (transurethral). This is accomplished by a small rod which is inserted through the urethral tube in the penis to the prostate gland. The rod has an electrical device that literally burns away the tissue in that area. This process is called electrocautery. Essentially the doctor makes a much larger opening by boring out excess tissue from the prostate. This excess tissue is flushed out of the penis and bladder through the specialized instrument. The amount of tissue that has to be bored out depends on the size of both the prostate gland and the opening that's left after it's enlarged. This process eliminates the necessity of making an incision through the abdomen. However, under certain conditions, such as an exceptionally large prostate, this procedure is impossible and abdominal surgery is required.

The small muscular sphincters that control the flow of urine out of the bladder are located at the region of the prostate gland. These little muscle sphincters are important since they prevent seepage of urine from the bladder. They automatically open for urination, and close automatically at the time of orgasm so that seminal fluid cannot enter the bladder. When the prostate is reamed out in the center, the terminal ends of the nerves in this area causing these muscles to function are cut, and usually the function of the muscle is affected. The problems caused by this approach, however, are commonly less severe than other methods of removing the prostate gland. Sometimes if the prostate is exceptionally large or for other reasons it may be necessary to make an incision in the abdomen just above the pubic bone and by usual surgical techniques literally shell out or cut away the prostate gland.

The prostate gland can be removed through an incision made along the side of the scrotum between the legs. This approach usually causes more post-surgical complication than the other two methods and for this reason it is not used very often any more.

The tubes that drain sperm from the testicles attach directly to the outer layer of the prostate gland, and are not affected by the boring out of the center of the prostate gland. If there is total and complete surgical removal of the gland, the tubes can be tied off. Tying off the tubes in conjunction with prostate surgery is sometimes done to prevent postoperative inflammation of the epididymis (the cordlike structure along the round testicular body).

As far as prostate replacement is concerned, there is really no reason to do it and there is no procedure that has been developed for that purpose.

CANCER

Dear Dr. Lamb—Please set my mind at rest. We have just found out that my husband has cancer of the prostate gland. Does that put me in jeopardy? Will it cause me to have cancer of the cervix or uterus?

Comment—Absolutely not. Cancer of the prostate is not contagious and won't affect the woman in any way. It's one of the most common cancers that men have. Five percent of men by age fifty have cancer of the prostate, and the frequency of it increases with advancing years. In the United States 17,000 men die each year from cancer of the prostate. The problem is that it's usually not detected early enough for surgical removal. The cancer may already have spread to other parts of the body. As with other cancers, one of the best ways to protect men against cancer of the prostate is early detection. This means at least an annual medical examination which specifically includes a rectal examination so that the prostate gland can be felt.

The earliest sign of cancer of the prostate is often a small buttonlike projection on the back side of the prostate gland which can be felt by rectal examination. In the military services where rectal examinations are required annually in middle-aged men, the cancer is detected sufficiently early so that about half can be removed surgically. In civilian life the batting average is not nearly as good, and only about one in twenty men have prostate cancer detected early enough so that it can be removed surgically.

Another procedure which aids in early detection is a special blood test which measures the "serum acid phosphatase." In men fifty years of age and older this too can be done annually. This is an enzyme which is essentially restricted to the prostate gland but if there is a cancer and it has grown enough to break the capsule of the prostate gland, increased amounts of this enzyme are found in the blood.

POSTOPERATIVE PROBLEMS

Dear Dr. Lamb—I had a surgical removal of my prostate because it showed cancer. Thank heaven they got it all. Now my problem is that after they took the hose from my bladder, which was in for eleven days, I have no control over my water. I have been wearing a clamp on my penis ever since they took the hose out of my bladder. What causes this and how long will it go on? I am getting pretty discouraged. I wet my pants often even with the clamp on. If I cough or sneeze, I can't hold my water.

Comment—This is an expected complication after prostate surgery. The injured muscle at the outlet of the bladder which keeps it closed between urinations needs to heal and recover its function. The nerve endings which stimulate the muscle to normal activity also need to grow back. Completely normal control of urine may require many months. Doctors commonly give their patients instructions on exercises and training methods which help to speed up regaining control of normal bladder function. The length of time it takes for this to be successful varies, however.

Dear Dr. Lamb—Can a man father children after the prostate gland is taken out? My husband had an operation about two months ago and had the prostate gland removed. He tells me I don't need to use my protection, that the sperm goes into the bladder and comes out in the urine. Would you please answer because it is important that I know for sure.

Comment—I am reluctant to say that a man cannot father children, since after all it only takes one sperm cell in the right place to cause a pregnancy. It is true, however, that the ejaculation is usually backward into the bladder. This is because the muscular valve that shuts off the bladder is damaged, and the outlet of the bladder at the prostate gland is open. A man experiences a complete orgasmic reaction but the fluid runs backward into the bladder instead of out through the penis. However, if just one drop escapes in the usual fashion, it may contain enough sperm to induce pregnancy.

Dear Dr. Lamb—My husband would raise Cain if he knew I wrote you, but I need some information. He had a prostate gland operation several years ago and the doctor told both of us that it would be possible for us to regain our normal sex life, but that we would have to practice by trying it several times a week until his ability for sex returned. To make a long story short, after the operation he didn't feel like it and so we didn't practice it. Now we're unable to have sex. When we go to bed, my husband wants me to know that he still loves me. He feels around and then I am really interested in him and try the real way. He tries to get ready but he can't. He takes his finger and goes up inside me and I get satisfied. He still turns me on just like before, for I love my husband and would never refuse him anything. Is there something we can do about this problem?

Comment—It seems to me that this couple is already doing something about this problem. At least the lady is receiving sexual satisfaction, even though the man may still feel frustrated. There are very few men who really have trouble with impotence after a transurethral resection operation. There may be a little difficulty at first, but like any other case of impotence, confidence is an important aspect. A sympathetic wife and recurrent efforts solve the problem in many men. If the problem persists, the man should go to the doctor for a complete examination. If he is able to obtain erections at any other time, his problem is not medical and is not caused by surgery.

There are many different ways that couples can enjoy sexual expression, particularly if they are willing to experiment with something besides the traditional man on top in bed in a dark room at night. These other means of sexual expression are particularly important when one or the other of the partners is sexually disabled for any reason, and the couple still wish to have some means of enjoying sex.

HORMONES

Dear Dr. Lamb—Is it possible to obtain the new hormone,

267

medrogesterone, in the United States? I have read that it can be used to treat prostate trouble.

Comment—Medrogesterone is one of many hormones being studied to see if they can shrink the prostate gland. This particular one has been investigated by Drs. Robert E. Rangno, Peter J. McLeon, John Ruedy, and R. I. Ogilvie. They reported their studies in the medical journal, *Clinical Pharmacology and Therapeutics*. In their early studies they investigated the use of this hormone in older men whose medical history ruled out surgery. Preliminary investigations indicate that the medicine may be effective in partially reducing the size of the gland.

There are a number of newspaper reports about different agents that are under study. Some are called anti-sex hormones reported to be under study in Germany. With the amount of interest in this area, no doubt some medications will be developed that will be useful. They will first be reported in countries other than the United States, however, because the U.S. Food and Drug Administration regulations are relatively stringent about trials on new medicines in this country.

Dear Dr. Lamb—About two years ago I had a prostate operation and they found cancer. A month later my testicles were removed. Subsequent X-rays showed that the cancer had affected my spine. I am taking hormone pills and I have read in books and magazines that hormone products have the ability to speed up the growth of some kinds of cancer when used in a patient who already has cancer. Is there any other product that can be used instead of hormones in my case?

Comment—This is an example that a little information is a dangerous thing. There are a number of doctors who think that female hormones speed up cancer of the breast and female organs. Cancer of the prostate is speeded up by male hormones or testosterone, not female hormones. This is why individuals who have cancer of the prostate that has spread to other parts of the body are often castrated. This removes

268

the major source of testosterone. The hormone pills that are then given are not testosterone but female hormones, or estrogens. We do know that the prostate gland develops under the influence of testosterone—if there is no testosterone available, the prostate gland does not develop. This can be observed in young eunuchs. Female hormones inhibit the growth of the prostate cancer and thus are commonly used. Some doctors treat men with female hormones and radiation without castration.

Dear Dr. Lamb—Would male hormones, if taken, be dangerous to the prostate gland or have any dangerous effects?

Comment—Possibly. We do know that the development of the size of the prostate gland is dependent upon male hormones. Removal of the testicles, for example, causes regression in the size of the prostate. Male hormones can also activate a cancer of the prostate. For this reason, as men get older, particularly if they have any evidence of prostate problems, doctors prefer not to give testosterone, or if it is given to provide it in small amounts.

PREVENTION OF PROSTATE TROUBLE

Dear Dr. Lamb—I have read that prostate cancer is aggravated by male hormones. Would a vasectomy help prevent this, or is there any way at all that older men can keep their male hormones from reaching the prostate gland?

Comment—A vasectomy has no effect on the amount of male hormones produced by the testicles. It merely blocks the movement of sperm from the testicles to the prostate. In other words a vasectomy is an operation done to sterilize the male. The testicles continue to produce male hormone which enters the bloodstream and is distributed throughout the body. Thus as long as there are testicles producing male hormone and a bloodstream to carry the hormone, they will be distributed throughout the body.

Dear Dr. Lamb—What is your opinion of the Japanese theory regarding prostate gland problems? The way it was explained to me, when a married man reaches the age of forty-five, he limits his sex relations to once a month. I can't see how a man and wife could adjust their lives to such a regime without creating problems. Does anyone really know what causes an enlargement of the prostate gland? We know that alcoholic drinks aggravate this condition, but do they help cause it? We also know that riding on tractors all day contributes to it, and that wearing a support sometimes helps to relieve the discomfort. Since doctors are of different opinions, I would like to know what your ideas are along these lines.

Comment—In the first place I don't believe that Japanese men at forty-five restrict their sexual activity to once a month. Secondly, there is no evidence that sexual abstinence effectively prevents prostate trouble. Evidence exists to indicate that sexual activity in the male increases his production of testosterone, but simple abstinence is not likely to decrease this sufficiently to prevent progressive enlargement of the prostate gland.

Inflammation of the prostate calls for some degree of dietary discretion—foods that produce irritating and acid substances to be passed in the urine should be avoided. They include coffee, tea, alcohol, and excessively spicy foods. There is some evidence that constant banging of the crotch area, such as rough riding on a tractor, can aggravate prostate conditions, but there is no proof that it actually causes prostate enlargement.

Dear Dr. Lamb—I have been worried about prostate trouble for some time and although I don't have difficulty now, I would like to take some action while I am still healthy to eliminate the problem. I believe that male hormones are the real problem and since I am married and have several grandchildren, I don't see any reason that I shouldn't do something about it. In short, could

I be castrated to prevent prostate trouble? If so, where would I go to get the job done? I don't need my testicles any more, and I'd rather do without them than to develop prostate trouble.

Comment—This is a rather drastic preventive approach. It might work but it isn't being done for that purpose. In a similar letter from another man, he offered to donate his testicles to the medical center or make them available to someone for transplant. Interestingly enough, years ago human testicle transplants were attempted, but there was considerable difficulty in obtaining an adequate supply. Taking female hormones might also prevent prostate trouble. However, both of these procedures could significantly alter a man's sex life. There has not been sufficient interest by men in these procedures to have stimulated any great effort to assess their effectiveness. The few studies of castrates that have been performed indicate that prostatic enlargement was not always prevented by the operation.

XV

Sex in Later Years

ONE OF THE LAST BASTIONS of sexual repression in American society is directed toward sexual activity in older people.

The idea that grandma and grandpa would go to bed for any other reason than to sleep, read the newspaper, or watch TV is beyond the comprehension of some younger people. Indeed, even some older people have been conditioned to this attitude. This attitude that sex should end with the middle years is not shared in other cultures. For example, in Korea, in a Confucian household where the elderly are still treated with respect, it is quite a different story. When the old patriarch begins to get irritable or nasty, he is provided with a young woman. This frequently improves his disposition.

In recent years there has been an increasing awareness of the sexual needs of older people. Studies in older people show that they do indeed continue to enjoy an active sex life provided their health permits and they are not unduly inhibited by social attitudes. Several studies indicate there is a direct correlation between sexual activity and good health. Dr. James A. Peterson from the University of Southern California believes that people are happy and healthier if they are able to express themselves lovingly. There is no more reason for a couple to feel guilty about having sex after fifty for pleasure than there is for younger people to feel guilty about having sexual pleasure before fifty. Once it is accepted that sex can be used for something besides pregnancy, age is no longer a significant factor from a social or moral point of view.

History documents the fact that sex continues into later years. Sylvester McGee, one of the oldest living Americans, was known to have fathered a child at age 109. While sexual drive and capacity may diminish with increasing years, it is still present in both men and women.

As discussed previously, one possible reason that there is an earlier decline in sexual capacity in American men than in some other societies may be related to atherosclerosis, or fatty deposits in the arteries to the testicles.

DESIRE AND FREQUENCY

There is quite a variation in desire and frequency of the sex act in older people, just as there is in younger individuals. Many older people continue to have a healthy sex life in later years and have essentially the same reactions that younger people do. Numerous letters attest to this fact.

Dear Dr. Lamb—My husband and I are greatly worried about a problem he has had the last several years. My husband is seventy-one and I am sixty-three. We enjoy intercourse twice a week. His problem is that his orgasms are small in amount. Is this because of his age? Is something physically wrong with him? His desire for sex is almost as great as it was when he was younger. Is there any medication that would increase this amount?

Comment—The size of orgasm in men commonly decreases with age, as the amount of fluid produced by the prostate and the little seminal vesicle structures adjacent to the prostate decreases. This should in no way limit a man's capacity to enjoy sex, or the woman's capacity to respond. This letter, however, exemplifies clearly the continued enjoyable sex life of a man over seventy years of age with his wife.

Dear Dr. Lamb—I am seventy-nine years old and still have

273

a monthly urge, but it's under suppression. I have a beautiful lady companion but I feel that I must not touch her. She loves kisses and hugs but no further, which aggravates the situation. Our problem is such financially that we cannot marry. We live in a mobile home and visit each other. In the wee hours of the morning I have no one to put my arm around and love. It's a plague. We need each other and she is so nice and so beautiful, and she needs me too. I don't know how to put it, but the Apostle Paul said, "It's better to marry than to burn," and I do burn. Doctor, is there anything I can do about this problem?

Comment—This is more of a social problem than a medical one. Many older people do live apart for financial reasons even though they have desire for each other.

Dear Dr. Lamb—I am too embarrassed to go to my own doctor so I hope you can help me. I am a sixty-year-old widow and my husband has been dead over six years. I don't know what to do about my strong physical needs. Once in a while I dream of my husband and just when we are ready for intercourse, I waken and get so desperate for release that I am forced to masturbate. This has caused me to hurt so bad around the clitoris and surrounding areas that I get sharp pains and it hurts for weeks. What does a woman do for sexual release? Will this hurt permanently? I am so humiliated and feel so indecent, but I'm not. I just don't know how to cope with this.

Comment—This is one of the sexual frustrations of older people. The loss of a mate also means the loss of their usual means of sexual expression. Of course, the ideal solution is a new mate, but since there are so many more older unmarried women than men, this obviously won't work for everybody. No small number of women who have previously been married do masturbate for sexual release. The study by Kinsey and his collaborators confirmed this point. It is, after all, the second most common form of sexual expression.

274

Dear Dr. Lamb—I am seventy-five and have the same sex drive that I had when I was thirty-eight—every two weeks. My wife doesn't. It bothers me. What can I do to curb this desire?

Comment—This is the man's equivalent of the woman's problem in the previous letter. The same rule that applies to younger years applies to older years. Both partners in a marriage situation should try to understand each other's needs and help each other. This is one of the bases for a strong marriage.

Dear Dr. Lamb—When I married my husband he told me I didn't have to submit to his sexual advances. We were already in our middle years, but I wanted him to have what was his right. For years we had an enjoyable sex relationship and the narcotic effect produced a deep sleep. Now he's seventy-two and just recently he stopped responding to me sexually. This happened just after he returned from the hospital for an operation on his colon.

Now instead of making love to me he holds one hand over his sex organs when I approach him and won't respond at all. I grew up in a home where marriage was considered a sacrament and I would like to know if there is anything that can be done about this situation. I think he may need medical attention. I want him to be happy in our marriage. In marriage as in life generally, it seems more blessed to give than to receive.

Comment—Age and illness sometimes decrease the sexual capacity of one of the mates. This is another example that emphasizes the continued interest of the female in sexual activities even though she may be advanced in years. Her husband may be having trouble with impotence after his surgery and in relation to his age. He may be avoiding sex because he fears failure.

Dear Dr. Lamb—I want to ask if there are any pills in the

275

drugstore that a man can take who's over sixty-seven. We are both over sixty-seven and I am very sexy and passionate, but my mate can't erect. You know what I mean. I wouldn't let this break us up as I love him too much, and he's a wonderful mate.

Comment—American men in this age group often have this problem (see Impotence). A complete examination is the first step, for sometimes the problem has a medical solution.

Dear Dr. Lamb—There are so many things on sex, but never anything for much older people. My husband is eighty and I'm seventy-two, yet sex is our major problem. I feel I've had enough and he says he'll never have enough. He's recently had the prostate operation and continually wants to keep trying although he wasn't able to do the act two years before the surgery. The ordeal is just more than my health will permit, but he pouts for days if I don't give in. Am I doing him an injustice or should he adjust to this change in old age? We've been so close and dear to each other. Do we have to end up in this atmosphere of hurt and pouting?

Comment—Lots of times in older years the desire is there but the flesh is not willing. The fact that this man had difficulty for two years before his operation strongly suggests that he will not recover completely his capacity for full sexual intercourse. This, of course, doesn't mean that sexual play or just good honest affection isn't still possible. It is sometimes difficult for older people to accept change or acknowledge the evidence of advancing years. Emotional problems can be created by failure to adapt and in these instances professional advice is helpful, even if it cannot totally relieve the situation.

DIMINISHED FLUID

As people get older their sexual secretions diminish or dry up. It is a direct response to the decreased amount of sex hormones in the body and happens to both men and women.

Dear Dr. Lamb—Can you help me? I am sixty-three years old and still desire sexual intercourse, and when I do I get a very good feeling at the end and a climax, but hardly any discharge, just a few drops. I used to have as many as fifteen good squirts and it made me calm and I could go right to sleep. Now I get nervous and just lie there. It doesn't make any difference how the female acts or how hard she tries to help me, I just simply don't go enough to satisfy me. Is there anything I can do? Please don't tell me to save it up. I have done that. I have gone without for as long as fifty days, but it didn't help me to get a bigger discharge. I think I've led a normal life and not done it too often.

Comment—This decrease in male fluids is a natural result of the decreased function of the prostate and other fluid-producing glands. As long as the man continues to enjoy sexual intercourse and reaches an orgasm it really shouldn't make too much difference what the size of the discharge is.

Dear Dr. Lamb—We are a couple in our mid-fifties. Sex has been a natural part of our lives and we've probably gotten along better with this than most couples. In recent years we have had some difficulty because we've evidently lost the natural lubricant that we had when we were younger. We've tried several possible lubricants but nothing really seems to approach the natural. Maybe it's just old age. Anyway I asked our family doctor about it and all I could get from him was a half-joking question, "Hadn't we ever heard of Vaseline?" There must be many people of my age who could be helped by an answer a little more practical and understanding than the Vaseline suggestion.

Comment—The natural lubrication that a woman forms for sexual activity decreases with age due to a reduced production of female hormones. The dryness of the vaginal vault that results can cause difficulties with intercourse. Vaseline is not a good suggestion. There are other lubricants, however, which can be used and are perhaps more satisfactory. These are surgical lubricating jellies or other water-soluble lubricants. A popular one is known as K-Y lubricant. You may be interested in one woman's comment on its use.

> *Dear Dr. Lamb*—I have had dryness of the vagina most of the thirty-eight years we have been married, but have found that a dab of K-Y squeezed on my finger and placed in the vagina opening changes intercourse from painful to pleasant. We still enjoy our sex relations and both of us are past sixty.

Comment—This will not replace the natural lubricant but it is a big help for many people. Unless there is a reason it can't be done, a woman's natural lubricant can be increased by adequate replacement of female hormones.

> *Dear Dr. Lamb*—I have a problem but I am too bashful to ask my doctor face to face. My husband and I are in our sixties and have a good sex life, but lately I have been having trouble with climaxing. I'll go a couple of weeks without satisfaction and then he satisfies me some for two times in a row. Then I have trouble again. I think I need help. I read in your column where a woman used a vaginal hormone cream and it sure made a difference. Would this help me?

Comment—Although this woman doesn't say exactly what her problem is, it is probable that she is experiencing the drying out of the vagina that will occur after the change in life unless the female hormones are replaced. Because sexual intercourse can be painful under these circumstances, it's to be expected that the woman will have difficulties reaching a climax unless the problem is corrected.

> *Dear Dr. Lamb*—What causes itching in a woman's vagina and is there anything to be done for it? I have been told it's nerves and estrogen shots would help. But they say estrogen aggravates cancer. Is this true?

278

Comment—The dry vaginal vault that occurs in menopausal women can cause itching. The chemistry of the lining undergoes a change with menopause, losing its previous high level of acidity and the secretions that normally kept the vagina clean and free of infection. The lining is now more easily infected and irritated.

Regular sexual intercourse helps the vaginal canal to retain its normal size, but the dryness of the vaginal vault makes sexual intercourse painful. Aside from painful sexual activity, itching can make the vagina very uncomfortable indeed. Creams which contain estrogen, or female hormone, do help the vaginal vault in these conditions, as do pills or shots. In some instances an active infection is present that must also be treated.

The doctor can do a very simple test to tell whether a woman has deficiency of her female hormones. It's done just like the Pap test with cells scraped off the side of the vagina and stained, then looked at under the microscope. According to their color and characteristics, the doctor can tell pretty well if a woman has a marked deficiency in estrogen. Replacing the estrogen will change the characteristics of the vagina. The problems associated with the dry vaginal vault— itching, burning, and painful intercourse—are commonly referred to as senile vaginitis or atrophic vaginitis.

SEX AFTER SURGERY

Dear Dr. Lamb—For the past three years, I have been dating a very religious woman who is sixty-six years old. In fact we are definitely engaged to be married. However, from her overall course of actions in our overall lovemaking—we've never had a sex affair, since her religion forbids that until we are married—I have reason to suspect it isn't all religion that causes her refusal. In the course of time she's told me about all of her illnesses and operations, but she says those operations have nothing to do with preventing her from reaching a beautiful climax in the sex act. I am very skeptical

279

about this since her husband died quite a while before her surgery.

According to her, she has had her tubes, ovaries, and womb completely removed. How could she reach any state of satisfaction or a natural climax? Will you please answer these questions since I do not wish to marry her, even though she is a real honey, if she can't carry through the natural bed partner act. I'm sixty-six but know I'm capable of complete coitus. She is a fine lady, but I still do not wish to marry her if she tries to fool me but will ease her out by other excuses and not hurt her or myself any more than possible. If I had money and was older I might understand better these assertions which I believe to be lies.

Comment—The fact that a woman has had her uterus and ovaries removed doesn't keep her from still enjoying sexual activity and she can reach a climax. Femininity and sexual drive are often maintained by hormone replacement. Thus there is no medical reason why this woman couldn't have an enjoyable sexual relationship. As to how she knows she can still reach a beautiful climax after surgery, that's a matter which rests between the couple involved.

Dear Dr. Lamb—I wish you'd comment on a man past seventy years of age who's had a prostate operation a few years ago and also whose wife died a year before, and because of illness they hadn't been having sex for several years. He said the doctor who operated on him told him it would not affect his sex life, as far as having an erection and an orgasm was concerned. We want to get married and I'm wondering what we can count on in our sex life, if any. I am about the same age he is and am very passionate. I have lived a clean life since being alone for the last twenty years. Would male hormones be beneficial to him? He says he gets an erection, but not like when he was younger. Is there any hope for us or is it hopeless?

Comment—Although American men's sexual capacity de-

280

creases in older years, this is highly variable. Most younger men eventually return to a normal sex life after a prostate operation. In a man in this age group it would be more difficult to say what the sexual response would be. It's a bit like buying a used car. If you want to find out whether or not it runs, you have to take it out and drive it around the block. But remember, sex under stressful circumstances isn't a good test. A couple improve their sexual adjustment with time.

SEX VARIETY

Dear Dr. Lamb—I have been married to my husband for over forty years and we love each other very dearly. Now for several months we have been scrapping with each other constantly because of a book my husband read. I may be all wrong but I regard it as trash and feel it was put on the open market for spicy amusement. I am ignorant of oral intercourse, and I cannot accept it at my age. Maybe I could have at a younger age. The book recommends this and it also comments on orgy parties and swapping of partners. I just can't believe this after reading it with my own eyes. My husband feels he has now been educated and it thoroughly disgusts me.

Is he sick or am I? Is this book good for older people, or is it just for young people? Or does it just cause trouble? I am not a prude but then I am not overly bright either. Is this book supposed to be educational for older people over sixty-five or is it just for the younger people, or was it just meant to be funny?

Comment—Oral sex contact is considered to be normal. Many recent sex books have commented on this and recommend it. Oral-genital contact also occurs among animals. I do believe, however, that it's safe to say that a large portion of older women are not particularly interested in this form of sexual expression. Sex between marriage partners takes two. For the relationship to be a pleasant one, both individuals have to enjoy it.

It's proper that marriage partners should discuss their sexual interests and experiment as long as it is not physically damaging or completely unacceptable to one of the two partners. In the latter situation, whatever the form of sex act, it would normally leave a lot to be desired for either party if one didn't enjoy it or frankly disapproved of the experiment.

It certainly is harder for older people to change their sex habits. People become conditioned in their sexual patterns and habits and are less interested in trying something new. Men often are more willing to experiment than women, particularly in sexual relations of this type. In short, oral-genital sex is not abnormal and many people do enjoy it, but not everyone.

ANTI-SEX WOMEN

Although there are many older women who continue to enjoy sex and have a strong sexual drive, there are a number of middle-aged and older women who are not at all interested in continuing sexual activity. This isn't too surprising, because a number of women don't enjoy sex at any age (which usually indicates an underlying problem).

Many women in the older age groups are products of the Victorian era, when it was still believed that "decent women didn't enjoy sex." The reaction of this segment of women was clearly pointed out because of an editorial change in one of my columns. I had answered a letter to a lady who complained that she didn't enjoy sex and that she was sore for hours afterwards.

Her letter also included information to suggest that she had senile vaginitis and she stated that she had a leukoplakia (a whitish patch) on her vulva. No doubt sex was very painful to this woman because of her medical problems, as I have discussed in relation to atrophic or senile vaginitis. Before an older woman can enjoy sex, these medical problems have to be remedied. In preparing this column, a newspaper editor removed the segment of her letter which indicated her medical problem. Quite naturally in my recommendation to this lady, I told her she should see a doctor. Many older women who are relatively hostile about sex were upset with this recommendation since the mention of her medical problem had been edited out of her letter. It produced a basketfull of interesting mail from middle-aged and older women who were basically through with sex. Their letters speak eloquently for themselves.

Dear Dr. Lamb—May I express my views in regard to your answer to the woman who had been married fifty years to the sex idiot. You say it's expressing love. Is the prostitute or the collection of dogs on the street endowed with more love than decent people? Do you call it love when a man gets his wife pregnant every year while he does nothing about it himself? Men like him are probably the type who have chased after every skirt and lusted after every woman when he was young, and now when no one wants him any more he gives his wife no rest and that's love.

When a man retires, he is retired and that is that. On the contrary, the wife has to work extra at keeping the house clean, extra cooking, extra dishwashing. There is the telephone, the doorbell, entertaining his friends and hers. There is the washing and ironing still, involvement with children and grandchildren and church and charitable organizations. There is the shopping, the wrapping and mailing of gifts, the writing of cards and letters. She signs these as Mr. and Mrs. and always both of them get the thank-you's.

Friend husband sits there with his continual blaring out of TV, radio, filling his belly and thinking of sex. Well, pardon me, he is just a selfish, inconsiderate, greedy man. Instead of the wife taking hormones, he should be given huge doses of saltpeter or whatever it is and if that doesn't work, then hit him over the head with a fencepost, so he will turn his thoughts from one end to the opposite end. You know what I'm talking about and I hope this will be put in print.

Comment—It's in print and what this lady's experiencing is not love.

Dear Dr. Lamb—You call this love? Those doctors, sex pushers obviously, call rape love too. One young lady that I know was married two years, already has two babies and a third on the way. Shouldn't her husband exercise some self-discipline? The doctor's answer was, haven't you heard of the pill? Yes, men have their fun no matter what. Poor women, no wonder they turn into ice. We've been married a long time too and our old age love is heaven on earth. There's plenty of love, the kind you don't know about, and tenderness and care but no sex making.

And from another letter:

> . . . but you, sir, are in a rut in your thinking. In this year of Women's Lib I certainly could accuse you of defending male superiority and the age-old propaganda of women's submission to man. I would rather hope for a line of thinking on a one-to-one basis, man and wife, where the give-and-take must be tempered to the individuals but not on any generalization.

Dear Dr. Lamb—I read in the paper about the lady who stated she was miserable after her husband made love to her, and you said she should see a doctor and perhaps take some female hormones. Well, you are not a woman and you have no idea what these old men do to satisfy their passions. They want to do something and can't so they take it out on the woman. They are no further ahead when they're finished than when they started, and therefore they are at you all the time. I would call this lust and certainly not love. All they want is satisfaction for their own body, no matter how they get it. I think they're the ones that need to see doctors.

284

And:

> . . . no wonder God regretted making man. Sex, sex, sex is the only word that men think about nowadays it seems and when I read your answer to this poor woman, I read between the lines. Oh, another man, and he's a doctor. He's afraid when he approaches advancing years his sex life will dwindle. I have news for you, boy, it will. That answer that you gave her that her husband loves her so much is "bullshit" from way back.

Dear Dr. Lamb—If you think that a woman married for fifty years to a man whose every waking thought is about sex who has been pummeled, poked, and pried at with little or no concern for her feelings, who has learned to dread the night and even the day, has any illusions that her husband is motivated by love for her, you are sadly mistaken. Perhaps you should come back next time as a woman and marry such a man. I wonder how you would feel about having your body not regarded as your own, but merely as a vessel for the pleasure of an inconsiderate, clumsy bore. You might not be so flip about wishing he would sublimate some of his sex drive with golf, gardening, checkers, or something.

And:

> . . . shame on you for telling this poor soul that it was love after being punched for fifty years. Do you think she believes he loved her? If he loved her, he would give her a rest. You have never been under a hog, have you? Well, I have, for over fifty-two years. There is not an inch of my body that is not sore due to my old hog. Would Jesus Christ call an old hog like that love? The old fool just wanted to empty out his old bag in that poor woman.

And finally:

> . . . unless both parties are agreeable, I think sex after fifty is unnecessary, at least for the woman, and disgusting, at least if more than once a month.
>
> Our lives should be a balance of all good. Maybe if he took his wife golfing or played cards or went fishing with her and they had a little fun together, he might get a bit of a spark from his old gal. That's the trouble with American men. They don't want to work at their lovemaking. Just "slap it at 'em, wham, bam, and away he goes."

Comment—These letters tell quite a story, and it's doubtful if very many of these women would be helped with female hormones in any amount.

XVI

Discharge and Hygiene

IT SEEMS TO BE AN AMERICAN TRAIT to be exceptionally concerned about cleanliness. Unfortunately, the term "clean" is sometimes confused with the term "smell." Odors are often unrelated to cleanliness. A fragrant smell sometimes masks the presence of many harmful germs, and on the other hand an unpleasant odor from certain chemicals may be totally free of germs. There are natural odors around the sex organs. That's the way both male and female bodies are built. Many of these odors are caused by specialized skin glands, which at one time served for sexual identification.

As clear evidence of American women's preoccupation with "feminine hygiene" and the success of modern advertising, in a little over two years time the hygiene spray market increased over $18,000,000 annually. In addition to the simple problem of odors, women have good reason to be concerned about vaginal discharge, vaginal itching, and other evidences of vaginal infection. There are many causes for vaginal discharge besides an infection. A cervix which is slightly torn during delivery may cause an increased amount of secretion in the vagina. Young girls, even before they start their menstrual periods, have increased secretions. These are the natural lubricants and since they are acid, they maintain a level of acidity in the vaginal area to protect it from bacteria and infections. If all this material is washed away, it may actually make the vagina more susceptible to infections. Excessive douching may increase a vaginal discharge rather than eliminate it. The heavy discharge of very young girls decreases and becomes less noticeable with age. This discharge in young women is white or clear and essentially odorless. Sometimes it develops a brownish cast as it dries.

Women in their childbearing years in particular are susceptible to vaginal infections. Probably over 30 percent of American women have this problem intermittently. There are mainly two types of common infections. One of these is a yeast infection, sometimes called fungus or monilia. It may cause itching and discharge. The other common infection is trichomoniasis, a particularly difficult little organism.

Of course other infections, including gonorrhea, can cause a discharge. Any infection of the vagina will cause congestion or increased blood supply to that area, which increases the vaginal discharge.

In older years, as the female hormones are lost, the acidity of the vagina is lost and it loses its normal protective mechanisms. In this case the vagina is more susceptible to infection by bacteria that normally would be unable to live there. (The problem of normal discharge in young women and the problem of atrophic vaginitis have been discussed in earlier chapters.)

VULVA

With the advent of sprays and "feminine hygiene" there have been many letters from readers who have had difficulties. This is a typical note.

Dear Dr. Lamb—Could you tell me if feminine deodorant sprays are safe to use. I have an irritation and was wondering if that could be the cause.
Comment—Yes, it can be the cause. When the vulva is irritated or inflamed, it is called vulvitis. The lips of the vulva can become markedly swollen, but when the vulva is tested for an infection there isn't any.

The degree of sensitivity to chemicals and sprays varies from woman to woman.

Medical World News, in an article on complications aris-
ing from the use of vaginal sprays, quoted an ex-customer
who reported that after only twenty-four hours of using a
spray, she had open sores with the most severe pain she had
ever experienced. She said that even childbirth didn't begin
to compare with the pain. The magazine went on to quote a
Manhattan gynecologist who estimated that 10 percent of
the women who used these sprays had difficulties. He recommended that women concerned with feminine hygiene limit
their efforts to mild soap and water. Cases exemplifying infections caused by sprays have been reported in the *Journal
of the American Medical Association* and in *Obstetrics and
Gynecology.*

Even so, these sprays are increasing in number. Dr. Bernard Kaye at the University of Illinois, commenting on this
problem and the variety of products available, talked about
one that was available in the flavor of mint frappé with the
fragrance of honeysuckle and "guaranteed to contain no
cyclamates." One of my obstetrician friends tells me that he
feels the upsurge in interest in "feminine hygiene" is directly
related to the upsurge in interest in oral-genital sex activities.
The sprays, however, are not the only causes for vaginal irritation.

Dear Dr. Lamb—I would like very much to have some in-
    formation on the dye used in pantyhose. Since I have
    been wearing them constantly for work, I have noticed
    an irritation around the vagina. I stop wearing them
    for a period of three to four days and this goes away
    and only returns when I resume wearing the panty-
    hose. Could this be the dye? I have washed them
    thoroughly and I still have this problem.

Comment—Pantyhose and any tight undergarments
frequently contribute to irritation of the vulva. I was amused
by one letter from a lady who had long ago learned the importance of clothing in causing irritation of the vulva.

Dear Dr. Lamb—To make a long story short, a sister of

mine doctored for years with this problem, trying to get relief. After many trips to the doctor and inserting ointments and huge tablets, the doctor told her she was allergic to nylon and she made the change to cotton undergarments and had no more trouble. My daughter had the same problem and I passed on the advice to her, and it cured her difficulties. I passed the word on to a lady in Texas and she is very happy that she was helped. In many stores you can purchase very pretty, colorful flowered cotton underclothes that no one should be ashamed to show.

Comment—Yes, and women who have irritation of the vulva and vaginal discharge would be well advised to wear loose-fitting cotton underwear. Tight-fitting underwear or pantyhose can be a cause of vaginal odor. Dr. Kaye claims that vulva irritation due to nylon panties or panty girdles is much more common than is generally realized. Women often have to pay a price for these feminine artifices, and the old-fashioned girl derived some benefit from her loose-fitting cotton garments.

VAGINAL DISCHARGE

Any woman who has a persistent discharge, one for which there is no explanation, one with particularly bad odor, or one which is colored yellowish or greenish rather than a clear or creamy color should seek advice from a physician. An examination will be necessary to determine exactly what is causing the discharge. Some of these can be due to trichomoniasis.

Dear Dr. Lamb—Would you please say something about trichomoniasis. What are its causes and why does it constantly recur? If the man is not circumcised, does he carry this and spread it to his wife? What is the best medicine for a woman and for the man?

Comment—Trichomoniasis is caused by an organism belonging to the same family that causes an amebic infection of the digestive tract or colon. It may also inhabit the lower intestinal tract and infect the vagina and the bladder. It can cause itching, burning, and discharge. Sometimes it's difficult to treat. In the past, many physicians treated it with douches. More recently, it is treated by medicines.

Because it involves more than the vaginal vault, frequently involving the bladder as well, simple douching usually will not eliminate the organisms. Successful treatment usually requires oral medication.

If the male also has the infection, it can be ping-ponged back and forth between the man and woman. Circumcised as well as uncircumcised men can carry the infection. Treating the woman alone will not protect her from a recurrence. Usually, if either one of a couple who are cohabiting have the infection, both should be treated.

In the past inadequate medicines made this infection difficult to cure. One of the better medicines now available is called Flagyl. With both partners taking this medicine for a period of ten days, the infection can usually be eradicated. Another reason for failure in treatment of vaginal infections of any type is the habit women have of only taking a treatment until their symptoms disappear. Treatment has to be continued long enough to completely eradicate the problem. This usually means continuing it for a considerable period of time after symptoms have stopped if one is using a douche, and for the full period of time prescribed by the doctor if one is using oral medicines. Failure to carry out the full treatment program means that organisms may still be present in the bowel or in the bladder, and reinfection is just a matter of time.

Dear Dr. Lamb—I am writing you about the problem I have been having for some time. I went to a doctor and he calls it a yeast infection. He has prescribed different things, but I cannot get rid of it. I get raw in the groin and it itches, sometimes quite a bit. It makes me awfully uncomfortable. Is there anything you can suggest for me to use?

Comment—Yeast infections, monilia, are entirely different from trichomoniasis and the treatment is also entirely different. Medicated douches, including vinegar douches, are often used in this instance. These too must be continued for quite some length of time after the symptoms have disappeared. The yeast fungus, or monilia, infections are particularly apt to occur if there is sugar in the urine. After all it is the yeast organisms that ferment sugar when the opportunity is available, and sugar in the urine provides the opportunity. For this reason, diabetics are particularly susceptible to yeast infections, but certainly not all women who have yeast infections have diabetes. Most doctors, however, will check a woman to be sure she doesn't have diabetes as a contributing factor to persistent or recurrent yeast infections.

Dear Dr. Lamb—I have had monilia, and although I am over it, I live in constant fear of this. Can it turn to cancer? I am afraid to have intercourse for fear it will start up again. Please answer my question as this is ruining my marriage, and also my life, worrying about it.

Comment—While a yeast infection can be extremely disagreeable, it cannot be transmitted back and forth between man and wife like trichomoniasis. It will not be reactivated by intercourse and it does not turn into cancer. Obviously, while the infection is present and the vaginal vault is irritated, it can significantly interfere with the woman's enjoyment of sex.

Dear Dr. Lamb—I would like some information on infections of the vagina. Could a vaginal infection cause any type of birth defect if a mother had it at the time she got pregnant?

Comment—No, the infection won't. However, for some of the medicines used to treat trichomoniasis in particular, there is incomplete information on what the effects are in the early months of pregnancy. For this reason, some doctors prefer not to use some of these medicines in the first three months of pregnancy in treating a woman who has a vaginal infection.

292

XVII

Venereal Disease

ALTHOUGH FOR A TIME venereal disease seemed to be under control in the United States and some optomists even predicted its disappearance, in the early 1960s it suddenly increased. In recent times it has reached epidemic proportions. Gonorrhea is the most common reportable contagious disease in the United States. Only the cold and related respiratory infections are more common, and these are not reported to the Public Health Service.

Venereal disease is defined as a disease caused by or propagated by sexual intercourse, but this definition is not entirely accurate because one can be infected with syphilis without having sexual intercourse.

Venereal disease has long been a scourge of mankind. Those who have it are in select company. The various notables it has infected include Caesar and Cleopatra, Napoleon, Catherine the Great, Goethe, Keats and Schubert.

The two common venereal diseases are gonorrhea and syphilis. Initially they were easily controlled with minimal amounts of penicillin. In adequate amounts, penicillin is still a very useful medicine in treating these diseases. Many authorities blame the pill for the increase in venereal disease. The pill is associated with a greater degree of sexual permissiveness. Also, individuals using the pill feel safe from pregnancy and do not give very much consideration to the problem of being safe from venereal disease.

Nature protects a woman from venereal disease by the natural acidity of the vagina during the childbearing years. The vagina of a woman on the pill will actually lose its acidity, causing her to be at least twice as susceptible to gonorrhea as she would be if not on the pill.

The statistics for the rate of infections for venereal disease in the United States dramatically show the sudden upsurge of the problem. In 1957 there were only 130 cases of gonorrhea for every 100,000 people. In 1971 this had increased to 308 for 100,000 people. In a similar fashion in 1957 there were only 4 cases of syphilis per 100,000, while in 1971 the rate had tripled to 12 cases for 100,000 people. In addition to the increase in gonorrhea and syphilis, the crab louse has been on the increase too. It is not surprising that there has been an upsurge of letters inquiring about venereal disease.

GONORRHEA

The National Center for Disease Control in Atlanta estimated that two million people in the United States were treated for gonorrhea in 1970. In various clinics around the country where women patients were routinely examined for gonorrhea, one out of ten were found to be infected.

Dear Dr. Lamb—I have a problem and have no place to go to get help. My symptoms are a discharge of pus which comes from my sex organs and burning or itching when I urinate. I believe I have gonorrhea. I've read about this disease in medical books which states it can be cured by penicillin. I would like to get it taken care of, but I can't go to our family doctor because he would tell my parents and they would have a fit. I went to a doctor I didn't know and he told me he couldn't help me until I brought one of my parents in because I wasn't twenty-one (I'm eighteen). Is there anyplace I can go for treatment without my parents finding out? Will it cost a lot of money and what tests will they run on me?

Comment—This young man's symptoms are fairly typical of gonorrhea. The disorder usually strikes a few days after sexual intercourse. Burning on urination is one of the first signs, because the infection irritates the lining of the urethral tube. Thereafter, a discharge is frequently noted. Otherwise, the individual may feel reasonably well.

Many young people are faced with the problem of obtaining medical help without parental knowledge. A good many of them do not realize that in most states the doctor can treat them without talking to their parents. As of 1971, the only states with laws requiring the physician to inform the parents he was treating a minor for venereal disease are Arizona, Mississippi, Wisconsin, and Wyoming. In addition, although Idaho, Mississippi, New Hampshire, South Carolina, Vermont, and Virginia have no laws permitting minors to be treated without parental knowledge, it is permitted under a ruling by the Attorney General. There is some difference in wording of the laws in the different states as to what constitutes an eligible minor, but in most states it is now possible for a minor to be treated for venereal disease without his parents' knowledge.

The other choice, and perhaps the best one, is for an individual who suspects he might have venereal disease to go to the local health department. They are authorized to provide free examinations. Also, they presumably would be less motivated than a private physician to make a report to a minor's parents in states with laws that require such a disclosure. Of course, the health departments can be and are used by adults of any age.

As far as tests are concerned, the male with a discharge will have a smear taken of the discharge to be tested and examined to see if the bacteria that causes gonorrhea is present. In addition, it is likely that a blood test will be taken to see if syphilis is present, since it is possible to have gotten both from the same or different sexual contacts. A limited physical examination will probably be performed to examine for any external evidence of venereal disease. The tests are simple and not painful.

295

Dear Dr. Lamb—In 1965 I noticed a discharge from my penis. I went to the Board of Health because several days before I had contact with a woman; even though she was married I wasn't taking any chances. Well, at the Board of Health I was given several shots and told to return in two weeks. During these two weeks the discharge continued. When I returned to the Board of Health I was told the discharge was not caused by a venereal disease but to have it treated by a doctor, as any type of discharge was bad. This I did and have been doing so since, but to no avail.

I have been treated by different physicians in many different ways, but nothing seems to help. Now five years later I'm tired of spending money and stuffing my stomach with pills and capsules. That's why I'm writing to you for help. Please tell me what causes this discharge and if there is a cure for it. Other than the discharge there is nothing wrong with my penis. I have no pain when I urinate, or burning sensation. I've been married eleven years and my wife had an operation to remove her uterus. I feel I am responsible for that and very seldom have contact with her.

Comment—A man may have a discharge that is not caused by venereal disease. There are a number of other types of bacteria which are not transmitted by sexual intercourse that can invade the prostate and urethra and cause a discharge. A chronic infection of the prostate gland can sometimes be the culprit. If the discharge is not associated with any detectable bacteria, the condition is called "nonspecific urethritis," which means inflammation of the urethral tube from some undetermined cause. Continued and prolonged treatment is certainly discouraging but is usually done in these instances. There is no connection between such a discharge or any other aspect of this man's sex life and the operation his wife has had. He has been suffering under a needless burden of guilt for many years.

Dear Dr. Lamb—I am very desperate and I want you to

help me by answering my problem if you can. I am sixteen and afraid to tell anyone what's wrong. For two days now I have had a terrible burning when I urinate, not during urination but right afterwards. At first there was a slight amount of blood in it, but now that is gone. I don't know what to do. I am afraid I may have some kind of disease. Would you please help me?

Comment—This young man is concerned about venereal disease, but pain and burning on urination with a few drops of blood doesn't necessarily indicate gonorrhea. Young men frequently have acute prostatitis, which is caused by inflammation of the prostate gland. The bacteria in these instances is not the same one that causes gonorrhea. A definite diagnosis can only be made through an examination. Such an individual, even though only sixteen, could go to the local health department to obtain one.

Because venereal disease is so common now, young men with acute prostatitis are sometimes hesitant to see their doctor for fear they have venereal disease. In so doing, they delay treatment for an infection which may have nothing to do with their sexual habits and deserves early attention.

Dear Dr. Lamb—Recently I discovered my son, who has been living with me, has been going to a doctor to be treated for gonorrhea. I am sure he went as soon as he found out. I'm in my middle sixties and have never had anything like this in my home. I am worried and would like for you to answer some questions for me. At the time he went to the doctor his girl friend had missed a period and now thinks she's pregnant. I do not know if she has the disease too or not, but my first worry is about the baby. Will it get the disease at this early stage, and will it affect it physically? My next concern is for myself. I wash his clothes and handle his undergarments. Also he kissed me full on the mouth when I returned from a week-long trip. Is there a chance of catching this disease from this kind of contact?

297

Comment—First, gonorrhea in a young, pregnant woman can affect the baby. Any woman who is pregnant and thinks for any reason she might have been exposed to venereal disease should report this immediately to her doctor, so that a proper examination can be done and treatment started at once. A gonorrhea infection can involve the sac around the baby and can even seriously damage the baby's eyes.

Second, as far as living with a person who has gonorrhea, this disease is transmitted only through sexual activity. Kissing does not transmit gonorrhea, nor does handling an affected person's clothing, cooking utensils, or any of the other common aspects of living together in the same house.

Dear Dr. Lamb—When I was told I had gonorrhea, I looked at my doctor and asked, what's gonorrhea? After he explained I wanted to run and hide and forget about the treatment. Instead I took the treatment and didn't ask any questions. I was given three kinds of pills at different times and still the cultures were positive. Then I was given shots and after three months of blood tests, the doctor told me I was cured. I had gonorrhea for about nineteen months before it was discovered. I have never been to see a doctor since I was told I was cured. I've been afraid, or better yet ashamed. Can a person have a recurrence of gonorrhea without sexual relations? I would like to know, having had gonorrhea for that many months untreated, if my tubes were sealed off? How can I find out if it has left me sterile?

I am thirty-four years old and being that age and after having had gonorrhea, if I could get pregnant, do you think I could have a normal baby? Can a doctor tell if you've had gonorrhea after you've been cured of it? I would like to have a checkup and Pap smear, but I'm afraid our family doctor will know. He and my husband are very close friends. Please, who can I turn to and what can I do? I want another baby but am afraid if I have one, it will be afflicted because I've had gonorrhea. This has worried me for many months

298

and I thought you might have the answers for me. It might also help a lot of other women who've had gonorrhea and are ashamed to ask but keep wondering.

Comment—If a person has been completely cured of gonorrhea, they will not have a recurrence of the infection unless they again have sexual relations with someone who has the disease.

Women often have gonorrhea for a long time and are unaware of it. About 80 percent of women have gonorrhea without sufficient signs of it to seek medical attention. Although gonorrhea can cause a discharge in a woman, it may be so slight that it may not appear to be a significant increase over the normal amount of discharge. This is one of the problems in treating gonorrhea—the woman who has the disease and doesn't know it, and has no signs of the illness.

The longer the disease is present, the more likely it will cause an inflammation of the tubes which in turn will cause them to seal off and cause sterility. I should think the way to find out in this particular instance would be for her to abandon any means of birth control and make an effort to get pregnant. If she gets pregnant, she'll know her tubes are open. If she doesn't in the course of time, she should go to a gynecologist for a fertility examination. Of course, he will want to know about her previous problem. There are other reasons why women don't get pregnant besides blocked tubes. Incidentally, there are many reasons for blocked tubes besides gonorrhea.

A woman who has been cured of gonorrhea and gets pregnant has as much chance as any other woman to have a normal baby.

After a woman has been completely cured of this disorder, she appears completely normal and there is nothing to indicate to the doctor that she has previously had the disease. There is no reason to fear a regular checkup and Pap smear.

Dear Dr. Lamb—Recently I have been reading much through the media about new strains of venereal dis-

299

eases showing up among our young people since the ending of World War II. Some of these strains are reported to be very resistant to antibiotics.

During the immediate postwar period I know of several cases of gonorrhea which went unreported and untreated among some of the younger soldiers who worried about punitive measures such as periods of restriction, etc. There were also some who went to German doctors and were treated with weakened penicillin from the black market. I imagine that some of these cases returned home still infected. Could you comment on the consequences of a case of a venereal disease such as gonorrhea going without treatment, or with improper treatment?

Comment—There has been a lot of discussion about new resistant strains of gonorrhea. This is a question of semantics. What's happening is that a certain number of gonorrhea germs are stronger and more resistant to penicillin than when the disease was first treated with this antibiotic. The more resistant germs are literally bred by inadequate treatment. If a person gets a little bit of penicillin, it will kill off the sensitive bugs and leave only the strong ones. The individual then spreads the stronger germs. In essence it's a form of selective breeding of stronger, more resistant gonorrhea germs.

These germs too can be killed with penicillin, but it takes a much larger dose than is required to kill off the weak germs. There has been a lot said about the resistant gonorrhea germs from Vietnam. This same process of inadequate treatment is responsible for this. Penicillin is readily obtainable without a doctor's prescription in Vietnam. Therefore many people treat themselves inadequately. Some of the young men you spoke of in your letter may have gotten over their symptoms and continue to be chronic carriers. Recent studies have shown that it isn't only the woman who can be asymptomatic and still have gonorrhea. Sample tests run in Vietnam war veterans have shown that although a limited number of them have come home with venereal disease, about half of those have an asymptomatic infection without being aware of it.

Some authorities on gonorrhea feel that asymptomatic gonorrhea in men is one cause of the spread of the disease, and estimate that in some populations as many as 20 percent of the men with gonorrhea have no symptoms. This suggests that men should have a routine examination for the presence of gonorrhea whether or not they have any symptoms, just as is now advocated for women.

Dear Dr. Lamb—Over six years ago I had sexual relations with a boyfriend who was having treatment for an ailment which he described as similar to the mumps in his sex organs. He assured me it wasn't VD and that it wasn't contagious. I trusted him then, but now I have my doubts. I wonder if he may have actually had gonorrhea and I might be infected. When I was married and again when I became pregnant, my doctor ordered blood tests which he said were normal. Since then I've read these blood tests were just for detecting syphilis. In an article in a ladies' magazine on gonorrhea, I learned that to detect gonorrhea you have to take a culture test. Is that true?

Since I've gotten married I've had two blood tests, five pelvic examinations, three Pap tests, and a normal pregnancy of a perfectly healthy baby. Yet I suppose according to everything I have read, I could still be infected and not know it. Could this be possible?

Comment—It's not very likely that this woman would have an infection in view of the fact that she's had a normal pregnancy and in the course of five years has had no evidence of symptoms. Nevertheless, it is true that the blood tests do not exclude it, since the ones that are commonly used at this writing are just for syphilis. Blood tests for detecting gonorrhea are under development (and may be available in the near future). The right way to find out is by a culture taken from the vagina.

SYPHILIS

Syphilis is a disease caused by a peculiarly corkscrew-shaped bacteria. It needs a moist environment to survive and it can live a few hours outside the body if it's in a moist droplet. It is almost always transmitted by sexual intercourse.

Once the spirochete burrows into the body and gets into the bloodstream, it begins to multiply. Then within ten to sixty days, with an average of about three weeks, a small pimplelike sore may develop, commonly on the genitals of either the man or the woman. While this sore is present and in the early stages of syphilis, it is called primary syphilis.

About three weeks after this primary sore has appeared, secondary syphilis begins. The person will develop spots and a type of rash which may affect the mucous membranes, the palms of the hands and the soles of the feet. The rash, incidentally, usually does not itch. There may be tender lymph nodes, fever, and other signs of illness.

A person with secondary syphilis may often be hoarse and complain of having a sore throat. These symptoms may subside and the external symptoms may disappear. Then syphilis is said to be in the latent state. Syphilis is no longer contagious once it has progressed to the latent state, and the acute symptoms mentioned above disappear. However, pregnant mothers can still transmit the disease to their children in this stage. Within the subsequent years, syphilis can invade the heart, brain, and other parts of the body. It can be cured at any time, but if it has already damaged the heart or brain, this damage will persist.

Dear Dr. Lamb—Recently you had an article on venereal disease, and I would like to ask some questions. It is said that if a man in his early twenties has a pimple on his penis, he has venereal disease. Is this so? How would he have caught this disease? We have been married a year and he does not fool around. Nothing showed up on our examinations which we had taken

302

before we were married. If his pimple is not venereal disease, then where would it come from and how would he catch it?

Comment—The primary sore from syphilis only lasts a few weeks, usually less than three weeks, and it is not really a pimple. Individuals can and do develop a pimple on the penis, particularly on the skin around the shaft, for the same reasons that people develop a pimple anywhere else. It has the same significance. If there is any question of syphilis, the pimple should be examined. The doctor will take a little fluid from it and examine it under the microscope. If it is syphilis, he can see the corkscrew-shaped spirochete that's causing it.

Most blood tests for detection of syphilis are fairly reliable, although they are frequently negative in the very early stages, particularly before the primary sore develops. An individual could have sex relations with an infected person immediately before marriage and have a negative blood test and then show up with his primary sore about three weeks later.

Certainly it should appear before three months has elapsed. If a couple has been married a year and not had sex relationships with anyone else and both had negative tests to begin with, it is most unlikely that such a sore would be caused by syphilis.

Dear Dr. Lamb—Can syphilis be contracted through blood transfusions? An acquaintance of mine told me she had gotten it that way and I believe her.

Comment—It's possible. Surgeons sometimes get syphilis if they have operated on an infected individual and gotten blood on their hands. Most blood banks would not use the blood of an infected person, and I should think the chances of getting syphilis as a result of a blood transfusion are relatively remote in the modern medical setting. You can get syphilis other ways, though, including kissing an infected person.

Dear Dr. Lamb—Twenty years ago I was cured of syphilis.

303

What I want to know is does it ever come back? If so, will penicillin take care of it?

Comment—There are occasional relapses in treatment, but this is usually because the treatment was not adequate to begin with. In the old days before penicillin was available, this was particularly true. A person who was adequately treated twenty years ago would have been treated in the penicillin era and would be most unlikely to have a recurrence of syphilis. If he did, it would involve the heart and circulation and nervous system, and it would not necessarily affect the sexual system in the same way it does in the early days.

Syphilis can cause damage to heart valves or the large aorta. If the process is unchecked, it can cause a rupture of the artery. Involvement of the heart and arteries from syphilis has been relatively uncommon since the advent of penicillin treatment. As recently as twenty-five years ago, syphilitic heart disease was reasonably common in the United States.

Dear Dr. Lamb—In one of your articles a woman stated that she had contracted syphilis by taking care of a person who had the disease. I have always been led to believe that this had to be contracted through intercourse.

Comment—For syphilis to be contracted the corkscrew-shaped germ must be in a drop of fluid which comes in contact with a soft, moist lining such as is found on the inside of the mouth or the inside of the vagina. Thus for a short time after a person who has contagious syphilis has used glasses or dishes it is possible for this to occur. If an infection is caused by kissing, the primary sore is often on the lip and looks somewhat like a common cold sore (but don't go around diagnosing everybody's cold sore as a sign of syphilis). It is not transmitted, however, from toilet seats or doorknobs.

Dear Dr. Lamb—Five years ago my sister had a heart attack and was hospitalized. Her husband was elderly and blind, and I had to care for him until he passed away. He had syphilis in the third stage. The doctor who cared for him didn't tell me this, and I wasn't as careful as I should have been in his case since I didn't know that he had syphilis. Is it possible for me to have it and not know it? This has bothered me ever since I saw the death record.

Comment—The third stage probably means latent syphilis, which is not contagious. It's only in the first two years of infection with syphilis that it is most likely to be contagious. After that it continues to seriously affect the individual who has it, including the heart and brain, but it won't be transmitted to another person, except by a pregnant woman to her baby.

Dear Dr. Lamb—I am a twenty-three-year-old woman and have a small child. I have a terrible and embarrassing problem. Every morning when I awaken, I have a severe itching at the outer entrance of my vagina. I have heard that this is a stage of syphilis. I did have several small pimples on the lower half of one of my thighs a few months ago, but it has gone away. I don't want to say anything to my husband until I'm sure. What do you think this is?

Comment—I think it is a good indication for a medical examination. A great many things cause itching other than syphilis. In fact, the rash associated with syphilis seldom itches. It is likely that this woman's problem is not syphilis, but a fungus or yeast infection. Nevertheless, she deserves a medical examination.

Dear Dr. Lamb—How accurate is the premarital blood test given for syphilis? Can venereal disease always be detected by this test even if it is in one of the various quiet stages? Also, is the same test given to a pregnant woman? If you've had these tests, can you be 100 percent sure you're not carrying the disease?

Comment—These tests are really quite accurate, all things

considered. In the first six weeks of infection, they may be negative, but thereafter the batting average improves markedly. If syphilis has been present for many years, then the test may or may not be positive. If there is reason to suspect syphilis from years past and there are other signs of involvement of the nervous system, the doctor may want to examine fluid from the spinal column. This sometimes will provide the information.

Incidentally, the test is sometimes positive in people who do not have syphilis. Some other diseases cause this reaction and a careful medical examination is needed to make a correct diagnosis.

Dear Dr. Lamb—Before going to the service I used to donate blood all the time. While in the service I had gonorrhea once. I checked in with the doctor three days after having intercourse and he confirmed it. I received a series of shots and was cured. Now my question is, can I still give blood? It's been three years since I've had this.

Comment—The blood test that's done at blood banks detects contagious syphilis and is unrelated to gonorrhea. In most instances, particularly in the service, if a person gets gonorrhea, he will be adequately treated not only for gonorrhea but also for the possibility of having been exposed to syphilis. Therefore, I shouldn't think this would interfere with your being able to give blood in the future. There is no evidence in the blood of previously cured gonorrhea.

GENERAL QUESTIONS

Dear Dr. Lamb—I am a teen-ager and hope you can help me. I got myself in a bad situation and practically had intercourse with my boyfriend, but did get out in time. However, I am really worried. You see, my boyfriend just came back from Vietnam and now I am afraid I might have VD. I would like to get myself checked for it, but if I tell my parents they'd kill me and I'd just have to leave. Do you think you could tell me if there is a place I could go to get myself checked where they wouldn't tell my parents? Also please tell me what would have to be done for this test? I know other kids are scared too but don't know where to turn. We're afraid our regular doctors would tell our parents and we couldn't face it.

Comment—The right place to go is to the local health department. As is mentioned earlier most states now have laws that permit doctors to examine and treat minors for venereal disease without having to tell their parents. The local health department will check and treat people for venereal disease free of charge.

As far as the test is concerned, there will be a blood test for syphilis. The test for gonorrhea in a woman is done by taking a sterile cotton swab and swabbing out the wall of the vaginal vault; the swab is then streaked over a special material that grows bacteria to make a culture. If there are any bacteria on the swab it will grow on the culture. If there are gonorrhea germs, they can be identified. The test is relatively simple.

Dear Dr. Lamb—I read in one of your columns that a person can catch venereal disease by kissing. In our science class a nurse told us that the only way a person can catch VD is by having sexual intercourse with an infected person. Can you explain the difference?

Comment—The nurse may have been talking about gonorrhea, which is not transmitted by kissing and is transmitted only by sex acts. Syphilis, however, is also a venereal disease and can be transmitted by kissing.

Dear Dr. Lamb—The medical profession gave women, young and old, the sex freedom pill. Now there is lots of free sex adventure appetized by mechanical sex education. Now we men are getting propagandized to commit sex fertility suicide but there are many of us men experienced to the fact that the condom is still our best insurance against venereal disease.

Comment—Well said. The condom will not prevent all instances of venereal disease but it does provide a protective barrier between the male and female and helps to prevent the transmission of any germs. The fact that people began to rely on the pill and other birth control means and quit using the condom may well be a significant factor in the increase in venereal disease that has occurred in recent years. The condom provided some protection against more than just pregnancy.

Dear Dr. Lamb—As a mother of teen-agers I am concerned about the increase in venereal disease. From what I understand, it seems to breed in filth and dirt. What I'd like to know is how did it start in the beginning? Is it a virus that can be caught from the air when conditions are right? A person can catch the measles without being exposed. Has venereal disease been passed down through the generations? How did it start in the first place?

Comment—Venereal disease is caused by bacteria. Gonorrhea is caused by a round-shaped bacteria with many of the characteristics of the staphylococcus bacteria which is found on the skin. I hasten to add that they are different types of germs and cause different types of infection.

Syphilis is caused by a germ which is corkscrew-shaped. These germs thrive in moist human tissues. The syphilis germs multiply in the bloodstream in the early infectious days and then will invade the various organs of the body where there is plenty of good moisture and food. The gonorrhea germ likes moist slick membranes and will attack the membranes that line the urethral tube and genital tract. It can also be transmitted to other parts of the body and can even cause arthritis of the knee.

Physical cleanliness is unrelated to venereal disease. A person who is physically clean but has the germs inside his body can still transmit the germs during sexual activity.

Apparently both gonorrhea and syphilis have been around for generations. At one time syphilis was said to have been transmitted to Europe from the American Indians by the men who came over with Columbus. There is a considerable body of evidence to indicate its presence in biblical times. Gonorrhea has been known to have existed long before the days Columbus discovered America. Neither of these diseases is inherited.

Dear Dr. Lamb—All the parents seem to be concerned about their children having illegitimate children and are happy with the pill. It seems to me that parents are as ignorant about the dangers of venereal disease as their children are. Why haven't these parents been told about it? Here are some of the things I have read about the disease and I would like to know if they are true.

   1. It can be caught merely by kissing an infected person.
   2. The symptoms are sometimes so slight the person infected is not aware of it.
   3. Even if they are aware of it and go to a doctor, they may be allergic to the treatment.
   4. It can be inherited, which means that a virgin can have it.
   5. It can be caught from a partner of the same sex.

Comment—Syphilis can be contracted by kissing, gonorrhea cannot.

Gonorrhea can produce so few symptoms that 80 percent of the women who have it don't know they have been infected and possibly as many as 10 percent of the men are in the same boat. Some people are allergic to penicillin which is commonly used to treat venereal disease, but there are other antibiotics that can now be used in treatment.

Venereal disease is not inherited. It can be transmitted to a baby from an infected mother across the placenta, since the syphilis germs in the mother's body will just pass through the blood into the developing baby. These babies have specific characteristics that tip off the doctor immediately to their problem. Other than in the case of a newborn child, it is unlikely that a virgin will have venereal disease. This, however, depends on your definition of a virgin. If sexual foreplay causes an infected male to lose some fluid at the vaginal orifice, he can infect the woman even though he may not have penetrated her far enough to have ruptured her hymen.

Yes, venereal disease can be transmitted to a partner of the same sex.

Dear Dr. Lamb—Can venereal disease be transmitted through homosexual acts?

Comment—Yes. In commenting on this, Dr. Warren A. Kettener, at the California State Department of Health, stated that 12 to 18 percent of men with infectious syphilis named other males as their contacts. Only 3 percent of the males with gonorrhea named other men as contacts. Either a man or a woman can get gonorrhea of the rectum. Also, an individual can get gonorrhea of the throat from oral sex. With the increased popularity of oral-genital sex, this is somewhat more of a probability than it used to be. The tissues and membranes of the throat are more resistant to gonorrhea than is the vagina and possibly the rectum.

Many VD clinics are now doing cultures of the throat and rectum as well as the vagina and penis.

Dear Dr. Lamb—I am a young girl and have read every article on VD I can find, but they all give me the same story. Please give me and other people some real answers on VD. For females, does a discharge necessarily mean VD? If not, what could it be?

What are the simple tests given? Are there varying tests and how long do the tests take? How long before you could get the results? Are they expensive? There are many people like myself who cannot go to their regular family doctor or their parents' doctors. Where can we go?

How long can a person go with VD before the damage is irreparable?

How long should one wait once tests are started before safely having intercourse and not infecting another person?

Comment—It's encouraging to know that young people want to find out real answers, because that is the best way to control the VD problem.

Young girls commonly have a normal white or clearish discharge which has nothing whatever to do with venereal disease. Any infection in the vaginal or pelvic area can increase the normal secretions and cause a discharge. A discharge from the vagina is also caused in women in their childbearing years by an organism called trichomoniasis or by a yeast infection.

There are some new tests for detecting gonorrhea. The culture that is taken from swabbing out the vagina can be studied in the doctor's office. Within forty-eight hours any germs in the sample will grow—if they are gonorrhea, they can be identified. A duplicate tube can also be mailed off to another laboratory to verify the organism's identity. Blood tests for syphilis can be finished in most laboratories within a few hours. These tests can be obtained from the local health department and are free in most states. If a person has venereal disease, he can be treated free. Thus it is not necessary for a young person to see his parents' doctor.

The sooner venereal disease is detected and treated, the less likely it will cause damage. If gonorrhea goes several months without treatment, there is a good opportunity for it to have inflamed the woman's tubes and blocked them so that she will be permanently sterile. Incidentally, gonorrhea can do the same thing to the tubes in a man and cause him to be sterile. There is no specific time limit on getting treatment. The best answer is as soon as possible. With syphilis, the longer it is present the more damage it can do. Even years after the initial infection started, it can attack the brain and heart and as long as twenty years later cause significant damage to the nervous system, or the heart and circulation.

If an individual has any reason to suspect that he has venereal disease, he should abstain from sexual relations until he has been given a clean bill of health.

Dear Dr. Lamb—Would you please give me some information on crabs. I have been itching in the vaginal area for a couple of weeks and just found out I have them. It really scared me. I also have a white fluid discharge that I've never had before. Also I've not had sexual intercourse in some time. Is that the only way it can be transmitted? I understand it is contagious. Does it linger in sheets or clothes? What do they do to the inside of you? How dangerous is it if it lasts a long time without being detected? Does it necessarily mean I have a venereal disease?

Comment—Apparently there is a marked upsurge in louseborn infections. This is commonly attributed to the new culture of long hair and poor hygiene. One company which sells delousing products estimates that as much as 5 percent of the United States population may be infected with some form of skin parasite.

The most common parasite in the current epidemic is the crab louse. They are commonly transmitted by sexual intercourse and they attack the pubic hair. However, they are spread by bedding, clothing, hairbrushes and combs, and even toilet seats. The crab louse is a very small bug, so small that it almost takes a magnifying glass to see them. They invade the hair around the pubic area and may also invade the hair under the arms, on the scalp, on the eyelids and eyebrows. They live by sucking blood out of the skin. It's the bite of the bug that causes the severe itching, which is the main symptom they produce. They are readily treated once they are identified. They really won't cause anything except the maddening itch.

312

Doctors often prescribe a medicine called Kwell which can be used as a cream or lotion and massaged into the affected area and thoroughly washed off twenty-four hours later. One application usually eradicates the bugs unless there is a very heavy infestation and then it may be necessary to repeat the treatment two or three times at intervals of four days. Of course, all sheets, bedding, dirty towels, etc., should be thoroughly washed to prevent reinfection. Anyone who has crab lice is also looked at closely to be sure they don't have venereal disease, simply because sexual intercourse is a frequent way of spreading the crabs. However, having a crab infestation does not mean that a person has venereal disease.

XVIII

A Question of Clothing

CLOTHES HAVE OTHER PURPOSES than keeping the body warm and comfortable. They are an extension of the personality, which definitely includes sexual attitudes. They are a sign that a person is male or female. Jane Trahey, who reviewed one hundred years of *Harper's Bazaar*, stated that men, whether it was conscious or not, insisted on women dressing differently primarily to keep them in servitude. Clothing is often the object of a fetish. Although attitudes about clothing vary between men and women, between young and old, everyone does seem to have an attitude on the subject.

TRANSVESTISM

If you are a Kabuki fan, you will know that that beautiful young Japanese lady on the stage is really a man. He has probably been trained from an early age to assume the Japanese female characteristics, including walk, habits, and most particularly dress. In wearing female clothes, he is engaging in transvestism. In this setting, no one gives it a second thought. If he tried the same thing Saturday night on a downtown street in most midwestern cities in the United States, he would be arrested and treated as a criminal. Social prejudices influence both individual sexual behavior and dressing habits. Western civilization in particular has es-

314

tablished fairly clear-cut definitions of appropriate attire for males and females.

In recent years with many of the social changes that have evolved, unisex clothing has arrived. Inadvertently, I stepped into a swirl of human emotions in answering a woman's letter to my medical column. It was a simple letter, and I thought I gave a simple answer. She had written asking what caused a man to wear women's clothing. The man she mentioned liked to sleep in women's briefs and panties. In a very short reply, I had explained to her that the desire for crossed dressing was not unusual in children, particularly in the years when they were exploring and growing up. I went on to suggest that for an adult to do this, having in mind wearing women's panties to bed, was an indication of emotional disturbance and suggested that she should get the man to see a psychiatrist or at least a family doctor. I thought this a reasonable reply, since I assumed there was a reasonably high probability that the man was at least anxious about his habit or might even have deeper conflicts and would benefit from professional counseling. Imagine my surprise at the types of letters I received after the column appeared.

Dear Dr. Lamb—I am asking for equal time to answer your letter to the reader who asked what's wrong with a man who wants to wear women's clothing. You said, "He's sick and needs psychiatric care." I submit in the majority of cases you are dead wrong.

There are hundreds of thousands of normal men in this and other countries who prefer "women's clothing" to "men's," and put these words in quotes because who is to say whose clothing belongs to whom. Because the underwear is silky and has a bit of lace on it doesn't mean it's only women's. Men wore lace on shirts and drawers hundreds of years ago. Because it's a skirt and not trousers it's not exclusively feminine. Men wear robes and skirts to this day in some parts of the world. Because it's a nightie and not pajamas doesn't make it women's wear alone. Men wore (and still wear) nightgowns. I do.

In fact, I prefer dresses to pants and soft fabrics to harsh ones, but in our "enlightened" world of today, I certainly wouldn't be able to dress in my preferred fashion for fear of arrest and ridicule. I can do it at home, however, and do it with the complete coopera-tion of my loving wife who assists me in choosing many of my "feminine" clothes.

I have had psychiatric counseling also and was told I am a completely normal male with normal male desires and the transvestite quirk is only serious if I worry about it. He advised me not to worry. Do as I please in the clothing department as long as my wife approves, but not to try and change the world's mind by wearing them outside the house. One question I would like to ask, what's wrong with a woman who wants to wear men's clothing? You can sign me a well-"dress"ed male.

Comment—This man's letter suggests that he certainly is well adjusted to his habits. At least, he's not suffering from any guilt complexes about it. What he says about identifying clothing as male or female is true. Men did wear skirts until approximately the eighteenth century. Eighteenth-century men wore high heels, Romans wore togas, Scotsmen kilts, and finally men wore a form of trousers which looked very much like a body stocking. Jewelry for men was in, so were lace petticoats, and the ancient Greeks dyed their hair blond and set it in curls. Both men and women wore pants in China and Persia. It can truthfully be said that in centuries past the question of whether the man or the woman was going to be dominant in the household certainly was not settled by who wore the pants.

Despite these historical observations, I still think that an adult male with a desire to dress in attire worn by the females in our society needs professional counseling, if for no other reason than to adjust to his habit and be certain he doesn't have any associated problem. My opinion is not unique. One textbook of psychiatry (*The Theory and Prac-*

316

tice of Psychiatry, by psychiatrists Frederick C. Redlich and Daniel X. Freedman), in speaking about transvestism, refers to it as a form of sexual misidentification ". . . in which individuals have the urge to wear the clothes and in general to assume typical habits of the other sex. Transvestites invariably are very disturbed persons; many of them are schizophrenics, but the symptom does occur in neurotic character disorders."

Dear Dr. Lamb—In this evening's paper a woman had written in to ask about her husband's wanting to wear women's clothing to bed. This man is a transvestite and I don't think a psychiatrist can help him, as this man cannot be helped unless he really desperately wanted to be helped and those psychiatrists who have tried will tell you this.

I am sixty years old and have been a transvestite all my adult years. The only reason I do not have the desires as strong as I used to is because my health is very bad. My desire is still there and if I can somehow get my health back I'll be dressing again.

Comment—This gentleman signed himself as a local transvestite and sent me a pamphlet which included many interesting points. The pamphlet distinguished between the terms "sex" and "gender," stating that sex is determined at birth, but gender is something individuals learn.

According to this pamphlet everybody is part male and part female, with portions of their personality submerged. Men who have a desire to enjoy feminine things or feminine activities are quite normal and have merely found a means of expressing their total personality. The publication strongly emphasizes that transvestism is not equated with homosexual acts (which the book called homosexuality). Transvestites appear to be relatively sensitive about this connotation and point out studies that have determined that individuals who have transvestism habits have no higher incidence of homosexual acts than the general American male population.

This leaves quite a bit of room since many standard texts of psychiatry acknowledge that homosexual behavior involves 5 percent of the general population and "possibly one third to one half of the male population have at least some homosexual experiences, and 10 to 20 percent who have engaged in sexual behavior with both sexes regularly" (*The Theory and Practice of Psychiatry,* Frederick C. Redlich and Daniel X. Freedman).

The male "drag queen," or the man who engages in homosexual activity and dresses as a woman, has created the stereotype that individuals who engage in homosexual activity are effeminate (which they often are not) and identified the transvestite with the individual who performs homosexual acts.

Actually the phenomenon of transvestism is not fully understood. It's complicated by personality and psychological factors as well as social and cultural attitudes. There are cases on record of male children being raised as females as well as the reverse. Sometimes this is due to a confusion in the anatomical identification of sex. In other instances, variations of the problem can occur because parents really wanted a child of the opposite sex to begin with. It is probably best to say at this point that crossed dressing in adults is poorly understood, both as to what causes it and what it means.

Dear Dr. Lamb—I am writing you for advice and, I hope, your help. I am a nineteen-year-old who is really messed up. So you will understand my position, I will try to explain how messed up I am. I am the product of a middle class home and have an older sister and brother. Both my parents are reasonable but very lenient. Now to get to the nitty-gritty or the dirt. When I was very young for some reason I liked to dress up in my sister's clothes. I knew this was wrong and yet for some reason I was compelled to do it. Even though I felt guilty, I think I felt I would soon grow out of this phase, but I didn't and as I grew older I found it was much more exciting to masturbate while doing these acts.

Many times I tried to stop but it has become a habit and I guess I just wallowed in my self-pity, so the older I got the deeper I dug myself into a hole. I knew I needed professional help, but I didn't have the guts to seek it. Well, now I'm hoping it's not too late. You see, while I was having such a damn good time masturbating, my testicles were gradually shrinking to a size today of slightly large peanuts.

I am not a homosexual, yet I am truly living a nightmare which is all too real. I am turning into a frustrated paranoid wreck, and I am thoroughly disgusted with myself. I cling to the hope of being a normal man who can live a fulfilled life. Please comment on my position. I have tried to be as honest and candid about myself as I can be and would appreciate any suggestions or help. I have written this letter in an effort to see if I have any future worth living. I have written to you in an effort to avoid too much embarrassment by appealing to a doctor I do not know.

Comment—This letter speaks eloquently of the anguish of the individual caught in the compulsion to engage in transvestism. This young man identifies transvestism with sexual stimulation and the sex act of masturbation. No doubt he also fantasizes, as most men do during masturbation, and in the process has begun to develop a conditioned response in his brain between sexual response and wearing female clothing.

The anguish caused by his guilt complex is adequate reason for him to obtain professional help. If he is truly oriented toward leading a life of heterosexual activity, he needs to get his transvestism habit in focus and resolve the multiple conflicts he faces. It is not likely that his masturbation has anything to do with the size of his testicles, if indeed they are actually smaller than normal. Small testicles have no relation to transvestism.

Dear Dr. Lamb—In answer to the lady who wrote you stating that her husband likes to wear women's clothing, you stated that her husband was sick. Well, if he is, there are a lot of sick women, for eight out of ten women wear men's clothing. They wear men's clothing on the streets and public places and also appear on TV wearing men's clothing so most all women are sick. The way I see it, it is ridiculous.

Comment—In western civilization it's much more acceptable for a woman to wear men's clothing. The lady policeman wears a mannish uniform, or a pants and jacket costume which may be relatively masculine or more feminine. The socially acceptable freedom for women to wear a variety of clothing, identified either as male or female, makes the occurrence of female transvestism less identifiable. There are many historical examples, however, of women who engage in transvestism. George Sand, the famous author, is one. She used men's clothing and a man's name to frequent literary circles which in those days were exclusively male.

Dear Dr. Lamb—Reference was made in your column regarding the man who wanted to wear women's clothing. You say such behavior in an adult is a sign of emotional disturbance requiring medical attention. I fully agree, though I am in no way trained in your profession.

My problem is a lovely female relative near and dear to me who, at every chance she gets, wears my old shirts and pants and acts so much like a man I'm embarrassed. Yet, when she dresses for dinner or church, she's lovely. Is a woman like that emotionally unbalanced and could a psychiatrist help her? She is normal in every other way except for this one idiosyncrasy.

Comment—There may be nothing at all wrong with this young woman. Some women feel a sense of freedom from the restrictions of femininity when they don men's clothing. This parallels the explanation advanced that men sometimes feel a freedom from the demanding role of masculinity by donning the clothes of women. Whether or not there are

320

emotional problems attached to these habits can only be determined by professional counseling. Whenever women have felt more freedom or independence these waves in history are associated with clothing which more nearly resembles that identified as masculine dress.

Dear Dr. Lamb—Your article relative to a man wearing women's clothing has raised a question in my mind. I would value your opinion regarding hippies wearing long hair and sometimes women's clothing. This matter is commented on in St. Paul's first Epistle to the Corinthians 11:14-16. It does appear to me that this is a mental condition bordering on insanity.

Comment—The unisex movement in young people is analogous to the long hair fashion. It is just that, a fashion, and shouldn't be confused with problems related to sexual identity. Underneath the long hair, beads, and unisex clothing is frequently a sensitive individual with strong sex drives for which his permissive culture provides an opportunity for full expression. Many of these young men are more experienced sexually than their fathers were at their age.

FETISHISM

When young men's fancies turn to panty raids and they invade the campus dormitories, it is reported simply as an amusing news item. But if a young man starts collecting women's panties, it has a different connotation.

Dear Dr. Lamb—I don't know just how to write this to you. Our eighteen-year-old son has a seventeen-year-old friend who is an only child and boy. They have visited back and forth several times, playing chess and different games in each other's house. John's folks both work days, leaving John to fend for himself through the day. He has also had the job of doing his family washing each week at the local laundromat. I suspect this has something to do with his problem. Having no

321

sisters to gradually learn the "facts of life" from, as he would if they were in some stage of disrobe now and then.

I don't know how long it took me to realize my underwear was gradually disappearing. I have never had very many as it was, but when they got down to only four or five, I used every excuse I could think of. Perhaps I left them in the washer at the laundry or the dryer. I made sure each time I washed that I didn't leave anything in either one. But still my panties were disappearing. Not the cotton ones. Just the silky or nylon ones. I was down to my faded red ones, faded blue ones and white ones. John had to go to the bathroom and was in there quite a long time. After supper and he had gone I was getting ready for bed and reached for the panties I had tossed over the shower rod as usual, and had forgotten to take them down. They weren't there. I had washed that day and there wasn't anything in the dirty clothes hamper at that time but the dirty ones I had taken off when I put on the clean ones. I looked in the hamper and even the dirty ones were gone.

Well, this was too much. All the other times I missed my underwear came to mind and all of a sudden I realized that John had been there in the bathroom too long. I wanted to be positive before making any accusations. I searched every drawer in my room, looked in every possible place but couldn't find them.

I thought the boys might be pulling a practical joke on me and maybe they had hidden them. I told my son and husband about them disappearing and asked my son if he and John were being cute and hid them. He said they did not. Then I thought John might have hidden them in our son's room as a joke to make him look bad, but a thorough search of his room that night and a better one the next morning turned up nothing. I didn't know whether to confront John outright and ask him about them, or tell his folks, whom we had met and talked to a few times when taking one boy or the other to the other's house, but I did not know them well enough to tell them what I suspected.

I let it go, and urged my son to talk to John if the subject ever came up. I didn't see John for some time but made sure that none of my underwear was ever left in the bathroom again. Then one day here came John to play chess again and needed to use the bathroom before he left. I didn't give it a thought until that evening when I needed my nylon half slip and remembered I had tossed it over the shower rod. When I went to get it it was gone. Another search of my room proved that it was gone. Then I remembered that John was there again and in the bathroom too long.

John was a year older now and hadn't been there for so long I thought that maybe he had outgrown whatever the problem was. I didn't want my son to have anything to do with him after I first realized what was going on, but John didn't have many friends and neither did my son. He is naturally shy and quiet, but has come out of his shell a lot since going to work this last summer. When I told my son I didn't want him at John's house alone with him as they used to be but they could come to our house and play chess all afternoon and there wouldn't be any talk of two boys alone all afternoon, he didn't want to abandon John, as he called it, because John needed a friend and maybe he could get over it. Our son said that at no time had John made any advances toward him nor anything out of the way in a sexual nature, but I don't know, if he did, that our son would admit it. I was afraid to just out and out accuse John for fear the shame would cause him to do something drastic—suicide or something.

We recently moved to a new apartment and here came John to show our son his new car. My husband

and I were out in the backyard and our son was eating a quick lunch before he had to go to work. I told John to just go in the back door. They visited while our son ate and then both came out to the cars to leave when John remembered his glasses he had left in the house and went back after them. I had gone in and made sure I hadn't left anything of mine in the bathroom. The clothes hamper was out in the hall, as I had mopped the floor and hadn't left anything lying around and shut the closet door, made sure my dresser drawers were closed as the back door leads through our bedroom.

When John went back after his glasses I got suspicious and went after him. When I opened the back door he was hastily leaving our bedroom, stumbled over our dog and when I looked into our room there was my dresser drawer wide open. He hadn't had time to shut it when I opened the door. He got his glasses and started past me and I said, "What are you doing in here? Why is my dresser drawer open?" and he was as red as could be and stuttered and said, "I wasn't over there." I told him, "Yes, you were. I think you have a problem. I have known about it for some time and you should do something about it."

He just brushed past me and went to his car and our son went too to tell him good-bye, not knowing yet he had been up to his old tricks. John left and I told my son and husband what had happened.

Later I asked my son what we could do to help John. Did he know what it all meant? Did they ever study anything in class about such behavior? If he knew anything he should tell me what we could do to help him while he is young enough to help and before he gets into real trouble. I told him I kept watching your column but had never seen anything on this problem. What can I do to help this boy? What does this reveal is wrong with the boy? Does the fact that he has no sisters contribute to this kind of problem? Does the

324

fact that he had to do all the family washing have any bearing on it? Is it a sign of homosexuality and could our son be involved?

I am at my wits end. It makes me mad, naturally, and revolted, but more than that I want to help him. I don't know what might happen in later years. What the tendency for such desires are in later years. Whether he might attack women, maybe kill someone in a fit of passion—I just haven't any idea. I never did know much about such things and am afraid to ask.

Comment—As with most forms of behavior that are not clearly understood, there are numerous ideas about what causes a fetish. The fetish, or collection of some object, can involve panties, skirts, shoes, or almost any object. It is not necessarily a sign of homosexual behavior, as this mother has implied in expressing her concern. This habit is a symptom of an emotional problem or psychiatric disturbance, but otherwise these individuals are often normal in their other behavior and are not dangerous.

Freud theorized that the object of the fetish symbolized the female penis. In psychiatric theory, the early emotional development of the newborn child doesn't provide for sexual identification between the male and the female, and the male child assumes in his psyche that all adults have a penis. Freud theorized that the man with the fetish had not fully resolved his infantile idea of the female penis. This helped to provide an explanation for the observation that it is men who have a fetish and not women.

Kinsey explained the male predilection for this form of behavior on the basis that the male sexual experience was more easily conditioned in association with objects and he learned to associate different objects with sexual experiences. Dr. Robert Dickes, psychiatrist at the University of New York, equates the fetish phenomenon with the childhood security blanket. He points out that the pacifiers that are given to infants provide objects for emotional security and that sometimes objects in childhood and infancy then take on sexual significance. In this way, hair, undergarments, rubber objects, and other items used in the fetish center around the childhood arousal and pacification. Since normally the child is pacified with the mother's breast, the object replaces the mother's breast. Dr. Dickes further believes that the days of toilet training may have something to do with selecting an object which is "used." Even our sense of what is a pleasant and what is an unpleasant odor is a conditioned response, and when the child begins toilet training, he thinks of his stool as an object of value. In the course of a number of complex developments, odors then take on new significance.

This woman's letter suggests that the young man she is concerned about apparently didn't mind taking used underwear. Dr. Dickes also points out that the objects for the fetish are often associated with masturbatory pleasure which may explain why the young man spent such a long time in the bathroom.

In any case a person who has a fetish needs professional help. This woman really should be very proud of her boy because he has stood by his friend and not judged him on superficial information. Even if this young man does have a fetish problem, he may indeed have many additional qualities that would make him a valuable friend. All things being equal in this situation, he should be considered as a friend with a problem who needs help, with the emphasis on friend first and problem last. A true friend can do a lot to help a friend in times of difficulty.

Considering the nature of fetishism, there is little reason to suspect that this young man will do anything drastic later or that his habits would significantly influence this lady's son. It is only to resolve his own conflicts that it is advisable for him to seek professional help. It might well be that this woman's son would be the key to encouraging him to do this. Indeed, the young man might be more willing to accept this kind of help if he knew he was not being rejected by the people who meant the most to him.

XIX

Miscellaneous
Sex Questions

THERE ARE AN ENDLESS NUMBER of questions about sex, apparently about as many as there are people to ask them. These cover the entire gamut from the meaning of recurrent erections to the advisability of sex for heart patients.

ERECTIONS

Dear Dr. Lamb—Is it normal for a fourteen-year-old boy who has had no sexual intercourse to have erections of the penis all the time? They happen with no particular stimulation, and I am afraid that one day they will happen in the showers and I will be very embarrassed. What can I do to prevent them from happening all the time? I know that erections are a normal function of the body, but I don't think it's supposed to happen all the time.

Comment—There are different levels of sexual arousal and at the onset of puberty the level of sexual excitement in boys is particularly high. If the sexual tension is not relieved in some way, there are constant and recurrent episodes of sexual excitement. There are very few teen-age boys who haven't been embarrassed one time or another by an erection at an inappropriate time. The exceptionally high levels of sexual tension in the adolescent years and the restricted opportunities for sexual expression in our culture contribute to

327

the high incidence of regular masturbation in the teen-age years.

Dear Dr. Lamb—I am worried that my marriage will go on the rocks. I work at night and sleep during the day; as my wife is cleaning the house in the days she tells me she comes in the bedroom to clean and she sees my penis enlarge a great deal. She says it's always like that and it makes her very mad at me as she thinks I am fooling around with myself. She is very wrong in her thoughts, and we fight every day about it. I sleep nude but so do a lot of men. Could you please tell me why my penis enlarges like this? Perhaps this will help me with my problem with my wife.

Comment—Men constantly have nocturnal erections. This term means erections while sleeping, and applies equally well to sleep during the daytime. These are related to the brain mechanism during the sleeping state and are beyond the conscious control of the individual. They have nothing to do with masturbation. Incidentally, they also occur in men who are sexually well satisfied. They are a reflex response. Studies of brain waves have shown them to occur at the same time as the REM, or rapid eye movement, dream state. Men may or may not be conscious of their dreams during erections just as we are often not conscious of our other dreams after awakening. The erections during sleep may or may not be associated with seminal emission. If an emission occurs, then they are called nocturnal emissions or wet dreams.

Incidentally, what a person dreams about in this state, if it has a sexual content, is also beyond the conscious control of the individual. Who knows, it can even be about having a pleasant sexual experience with one's wife.

Dear Dr. Lamb—I have a very serious problem and don't know where to go. Every time my husband sees a girl or woman in the paper, magazine, on television, or walking down the street, no matter what she is wearing, he gets an erect penis. I've brought it up to him and he always says I'm imagining things, but I have been married to him for four years and I know what it looks like when a man is excited and he has a big bulge in his pants. I have asked him to see a doctor, but he refuses. I have talked with a couple of my close friends (husband and wife) and they said it just isn't normal for a man to have this happen. I've tried to ignore it, but I can't any longer. We can't even sit and watch a clean half-hour show without him getting me upset. I have an eleven-month-old boy who will be growing up much too fast to have this type of father with a sick mind to teach him what he will have to know. My husband is twenty-four years old.

Comment—Individuals do have to learn certain levels of control, but it is true that the male mind responds to seeing things which stimulate him to have sexual thoughts. Fortunately for the human race, one of these is women. The reason a lot of men wear relatively tight-fitting undergarments which "provide support" is really to anchor down a rambunctious penis which is sometimes short on social discrimination. If an individual has persistent erections, as this woman describes, it probably means he has a relatively high level of sexual tension, and it may also mean he is not getting enough opportunity for release of his sexual tensions. In any case, it is not fair to say he has a sick mind just because he's sexy.

VAGINAL CANCER

Dear Dr. Lamb—I read an article that said scientists had discovered that stilbestrol (the female hormone) given to seven women during pregnancy apparently caused a rare vaginal cancer in their daughters fifteen to twenty-two years later. What can I do to protect my thirteen-year-old daughter whose mother was given this hormone during pregnancy?

Comment—There does seem to be a relation between taking

female hormones while pregnant and the occurrence of vaginal cancer in daughters years later. Now that this information is understood, there may be considerably more caution exercised in using female hormones during pregnancy. A girl whose mother was given stilbestrol while pregnant should be taught to examine herself frequently and to have a routine medical examination at least once a year. She should particularly look for lumps or sores in the vaginal area. Early detection can prevent the problem from advancing too far should it occur.

BLOODY SEMEN

Dear Dr. Lamb—My husband is seventy-three years old and every once in a while he still thinks he should have sexual relations, and when he does his orgasm has blood in it. I am worried about this as I think something is wrong. Do you know what's causing the problem?

Comment—Interestingly enough I have received a number of letters about bloody semen. Dr. John W. Grimes of Duke University, in commenting on this, points out that this defect is rarely associated with a tumor so it's not likely to be cancer. There are a number of things along the genital tract which can cause it. Commonly the seminal vesicles are a source of bleeding, although it can come from a blood vessel in the dilated vas deferens tube of the testicle. Other causes include any inflammatory reaction, including prostatitis, a small stone formed in the prostate (these are not uncommon), hardening of the arteries in the prostate or seminal vesicle area or elsewhere in the genital tract that causes hemorrhage of one of the vessels, or any factor which causes congestion and distention of the prostate and seminal vesicles (for example, lack of sufficient sexual activity in young, sexually stimulated males). An examination is indicated.

ASPIRIN

Dear Dr. Lamb—One day last week my fiancé had a head-

330

ache so I asked him if he wanted a couple of aspirin. He said no, and didn't I realize that a man could become sterile by taking too many aspirin over a period of time. This sounded ridiculous to me but is it true?

Comment—Partially true. There has been some research work that suggests that if a man takes aspirin regularly it can function as a birth control pill. I hasten to add that at this writing its true effectiveness along this line has not been established, so it should not be used as a method of birth control. In usual, intermittent doses it is doubtful that aspirin will have any effect on a man's fertility.

HAIR LOSS

Dear Dr. Lamb—Eight months ago I had a baby and since then I have been losing a lot of hair. I understand this is common. Other women have told me this may be from contraceptives. I have just begun taking the birth control pill again. Others tell me it is caused by the pregnancy. My doctor suggests I try another birth control method to see if this will help, but I am somewhat afraid to. I am also afraid of becoming bald. What's the truth about this situation?

Comment—Loss of hair after pregnancy is a fairly common problem. Fortunately, it isn't permanent and within a year after delivery, the problem usually disappears.

The loss of hair is not caused by the birth control pill and this problem has been noted for years before birth control pills were in common usage.

CESAREAN SECTION

Dear Dr. Lamb—My first baby was a cesarean baby. He's fat and healthy. I would like to know if there is any danger of me having another baby. If I were to have another baby, would there be such a thing as having another cesarean operation?

Comment—The cesarean operation is merely an incision

through the abdominal wall and through the womb to extract the baby. Some women have had multiple cesarean sections with subsequent births. With each new section the old scar is cut away in both the abdominal wall and the uterine wall. A woman, particularly if she has had one or more than one cesarean section, has very little risk except from the possibility of going into labor. If this occurs and the uterus starts to contract forcefully, there is a chance that the scar from the previous cesarean sections may rupture.

READING PLAYBOY

Dear Dr. Lamb—You may not think this is a health problem, but it is to me. It's tearing my whole nerves apart and I can't have a happy family life until I get help. I am so disappointed. A few days ago I found out my husband had been looking at *Playboy* magazines and other nude magazine pictures. The magazines are hidden and he has to go out of his way to look at them. He is a wonderful husband at home and takes us to clean movies and places. I feel now he has had a desire for other women, and I am not the happy person I was. What does this mean? Should I get nervous medicine or counseling? Do all men do this?

Comment—Considering the size of the circulation of *Playboy* it's safe to say that a large number of men do this. There is nothing abnormal about it, and a husband who looks at nude pictures doesn't necessarily love his wife any less. Men and women both have multiple ways of satisfying their sexual drives. Looking at pictures, objects, or people that stimulate them sexually is common. A woman who wants to keep her husband sexy will not prevent him from obtaining adequate erotic stimuli. This young girl should be happy that her husband only looks. While one can be sympathetic to her naïve reaction, it does indicate that she has a relatively inadequate appreciation of normal sexual response and levels of sexual interest. She probably could benefit from some professional counseling. It might significantly improve her marriage or keep it from getting into trouble in the years to come.

DRUGS

Dear Dr. Lamb—Please help me if you can. I am seventeen and an unwed expectant mother. I want to keep my baby, which makes my parents happy, as they don't believe in abortion. Before I realized I was pregnant, some friends persuaded me to try marijuana for the first time. I didn't get very high. Now I am so afraid the marijuana will have hurt my baby. It was so early in my pregnancy. Will my baby be okay? Can you give me any information? I can't go through the next several months with this fear.

Comment—There is professional disagreement on this point. Some studies have suggested that marijuana can cause birth defects. Other scientists have disputed this suggestion. If used only once in small amounts, it is not likely to have caused any problems, but in general I think young people are better off not to take the chance. A developing baby is a very sensitive, delicate creature and his future life can be significantly influenced by what happens in the mother's body during the nine months that she is the custodian of his development. She owes it to her baby not to expose him to toxins, drugs, and medicines that may be harmful to the tiny developing body.

There is more evidence that harder drugs are apt to cause birth defects.

Dear Dr. Lamb—My boyfriend and I are planning to be married in a couple of years, and like most couples we want healthy, normal children. Will hard drugs as well as marijuana affect our future children? I haven't taken any drugs but my boyfriend has. He didn't do it often but when he did they were hard drugs. This scares me. He has quit drugs altogether. Don't get me wrong, he wasn't hooked or anything like that, but he was just experimenting with them and quit.

Comment—The whole story of how drugs affect the chromosomes or genes, and in turn affect children, is not known. The best way to avoid this problem is to avoid drugs. There is some evidence that taking LSD increases the likelihood of cancer of the testicles.

Young people may be interested to know that there appears to be a cause-and-effect relationship between the frequent use of LSD and carcinoma of the testicles. Dr. Leonard Ledick of Albert Einstein Medical College described this in two young men who had taken over twenty LSD trips, and then developed cancer of the testicles.

SEX AND HEART DISEASE

Not too many years ago patients with heart attacks were sentenced to a life of inactivity. During the six-week hospital stay much of the time the patients weren't even allowed to turn the pages of a book or even brush their own teeth. When the patients went home, they were given very careful instructions limiting their activity to walking about the house; gradually they were permitted a little more activity, but very few were encouraged to resume normal physical activity. This period of medical history also corresponded to the time when sex was even an embarrassing subject to doctors. Consequently, the patient's sex life after he went home from the hospital was often not discussed.

Since sexual activity significantly increases the heart rate and blood pressure, sometimes to the level seen while pumping a bicycle or walking on a treadmill, the patient's home life often centered around tiptoeing cautiously to the bathroom and returning to bed to engage in physical activity equivalent to treadmill exercise. There are a considerable number of cases reported—and many more do not get recorded—of men who have had heart attacks during intercourse. Women suffer from this problem less frequently. I have personal knowledge of cases where men who have left the hospital after being treated for a heart attack have returned very shortly thereafter in an ambulance with a new heart attack or even dead on arrival. In recent years studies of how the heart and circulation respond to sexual activity are a source of objective information on whether one should or should not engage in sexual activity if heart disease is present.

This objective data has led to recommendations of limited value. The difficulty occurs when these recommendations are taken to be general rules, for in fact *each case has to be judged on its merits.* Just as every person who has a heart attack is not able to return to full, vigorous activity, not every person is able to return to full, vigorous sexual activity at once. Thus, no one rule can be made which will apply to all cases, or even the vast majority of cases.

Recommendations for a patient's sex life following a heart attack should be based on objective measurements carried out in that individual. My best recommendation is that if an individual has developed his physical capacity sufficiently to engage in moderate physical activity for a period of at least fifteen minutes without developing signs of heart difficulties, normal sexual activities should pose no difficulty. If a person's physical activity is limited to the point that he is only able to walk one city block or less without difficulty, he is not likely to be able to engage in a vigorous sex life.

Testing is best carried out in the doctor's office, supervised by professional personnel. The individual can either jog in place at a comfortable speed or pedal a stationary bicycle after which (and preferably during, if possible) heart tracings should be taken to see what the electrical activity of the heart is like. Blood pressure and heart rate should be monitored while the individual is exercising.

If this can't be done, the next best step is for the individual to gradually increase his physical activity in the weeks after returning home from the hospital until he can demonstrate that he can walk comfortably at a reasonable speed for thirty minutes without difficulty. If an individual begins to experience chest pain with this degree of physical exercise, he is probably not ready to engage in vigorous sexual activity.

Investigators provide differing figures on individual re-

335

sponse to sexual activity. Some say that the heart rate only increases to 110 or 120 beats per minute. However, Masters and Johnson's study has demonstrated that in some people, heart rates may reach as high as 180 beats per minute. These latter heart rates are equivalent to the highest rates that I observed in studying astronauts and endurance athletes at the level of near maximum physical activity on a treadmill test.

Some investigators believe that men who have sexual activity at home are inclined to have lower heart rates and less stress on their hearts than those men who engage in extramarital affairs. For those who believe that extramarital affairs are immoral, I suppose one could say there is a price for such a man's wickedness. The studies may also suggest that married sex loses some of its excitement.

Dear Dr. Lamb—After a man has a heart attack, he seems to be afraid of sex. My husband is in his early fifties and has never been sick a day in his life. Before he was hospitalized he was a very sexy man and quite popular. We have had over thirty-five good, sexy years. After his heart attack he recovered beautifully, even though he had to stay in the intensive care and all that before he came home. Now our trouble is sex. He seems to have lost all desire for it. Is this normal? Are there some kind of vitamins you can give men in this age so they can regain their sex activity? I'm sure those movie stars who have young wives and go on having children must take something. He loves me at the door, kisses me, but doesn't attempt sex like he's afraid he can't make the grade. Only once in the six months since his heart attack has it worked for him. Is there something ordinary people can take that isn't injurious? Don't those big-shots take something regularly?

Comment—This man's fear after his heart attack is probably inhibiting his sexual performance. Fear alone can cause im-

336

potence or loss of desire. One of the most useful things which can be done for a man with this problem, if it's truly based on fear after a heart attack, is to demonstrate to him what his physical capacity is by exercising him in the doctor's office and showing him how much work he can do without having difficulties. Once he finds that he is able to perform physical activity that requires the energy equivalent of the sex act, it often greatly relieves his mind and he can return to normal married life.

Of course, a man can develop impotence or lack of desire whether or not he's had a heart attack, and the two may be unrelated. There are a few medical problems which cause impotence, including disease of the arteries to the genitals. Diabetes is also a frequent factor in increasing fatty deposits in the arteries and heart attacks, and impotence is often an early sign of diabetes. I should think any man who has had a heart attack and has impotence should be carefully examined for the possibility of underlying diabetes.

Most men who have a good recovery from a heart attack can return to normal, vigorous sex life. Since sexual activity does involve a reasonable amount of work of the heart, it is important that individuals who have a sex life also maintain a regular exercise program. The exercise helps to keep their heart in shape so that the sexual activity is not an unusual event. Individuals who do this are less likely to have difficulty with their sex life.

Dear Dr. Lamb—I desperately need help. Two years ago I had a heart attack and since then I have been afraid to have relations with my husband. We did try once, but I felt very nervous. My chest felt heavy and I couldn't continue. This is having a very serious effect on us. What should I do?

Comment—Women can have trouble with sexual intercourse after a heart attack just as men do, and the sex act in women also increases the work of the heart. This woman, too, needs to be examined in the laboratory to see how much exercise or work she can do before she has difficulty with her heart. This would be helpful in deciding what caused her to complain of having the sensation of heaviness in her chest. In some people with heart disease exercise causes chest pain. This is a sign that the heart is being overworked and is nature's way of warning individuals to stop. On the other hand, chest discomfort in a woman who's nervous may merely represent nervousness or fear. The only way to find out is by a careful examination. If such an examination reveals that the woman should be able to enjoy sex without difficulty, she needs reassurance.

Dear Dr. Lamb—My husband who is in his early fifties has an enlarged heart, plus poor circulation. He is totally disabled on account of this. Sometimes it's too much for him to even dress or undress himself. He is very much distressed at times because he still wants to have sex relations, but because of the weakness and heart spasms which occur soon after starting, he has to refrain from it. Is there any medication that could be given? We would try anything to save our marriage from going to pieces.

Comment—An individual who has heart trouble severe enough that he sometimes has trouble dressing and undressing quite naturally is going to have trouble doing any form of vigorous physical activity, including sexual intercourse. Even if the man assumes the passive role, the heart and circulation work harder up to and at the point of orgasm. It's true that some individuals can do more exercise if they take a nitroglycerin tablet under the tongue before exercising. The same would apply to sexual intercourse. Some men can take the nitroglycerin tablet without it interfering with their sex act. Even so, it seems to me that a man who has this much difficulty should discuss his sex life with his doctor who is familiar with his case. It may well be that until his heart is strong enough for him to engage in more vigorous physical activity than simply dressing and undressing, he should refrain from attempting to reactivate his sex life.

338

DOUBLE VAGINA

Dear Dr. Lamb—Is it possible for a girl to have a double vagina canal? If so, could it bring about any complications during intercourse or pregnancy? If not, what is the reason for a division in the canal?

Comment—Yes, this is possible, and a girl who has one usually requires surgical correction of the defect. This and other anatomical problems are good reasons why every woman should have a thorough examination before she enters marriage.

FATHER OF TWINS

Dear Dr. Lamb—Is it possible for fraternal twins to have different fathers? If this is true, are there any cases in history as far as you know?

Comment—Yes, fraternal twins are those that are born from two different eggs (ova). If one is fertilized by the sperm from one man and the other fertilized by sperm from another man, the twins would have different fathers. There was such a case reported in Germany wherein blood tests proved that the two twins were fathered by different men. The mother confessed that she had been having sexual relations with her husband and another man. Incidentally, although it was previously believed impossible, there is some evidence now that one egg can be fertilized by two sperm cells. This raises the possibility that a baby could have two fathers, receiving some of his chromosomes from each man as well as the chromosomes from his mother.

HAVING BOYS OR GIRLS

Dear Dr. Lamb—I have heard if you douche with a solution before intercourse, you can determine the sex of your baby. Would you know the solution and if this is true?

Comment—Yes, this concept was popularized by Dr. Landrum Shettles, obstetrician from Columbia College of Physicians and Surgeons. The idea is based on the fact that sperm

339

cells carry either X chromosome (female sperm cells) or Y chromosome (male sperm cells). This is what determines whether a baby is going to be a boy or a girl. According to Dr. Shettles, the female sperm cells will survive in an acid environment and the male sperm cells are less likely to survive in an acid environment. If the male sperm cells are exposed to an acid environment, they are destroyed, leaving a large number of female sperm cells.

If a couple want a boy child, they should try to deposit the sperm as close to the time the egg will be ready to be fertilized as possible. This way the male sperm cells won't have to be in the vagina for hours and hours before a fertilizable egg is available. This increases the probability that one of the male sperm cells will get to the egg and produce a boy. Of course, if one wants a girl child, the opposite technique should be used.

To try to enhance the effects, if a couple wants a boy, they refrain from intercourse for several days until just at the time of ovulation, using the temperature curves that have been discussed earlier to help determine when ovulation occurs. Then just preceding intercourse, the woman should douche using two tablespoons of baking soda to a quart of water. The solution should be allowed to stand for about a quarter of an hour before using it, to be sure all the soda has been dissolved. The baking soda will neutralize the normal acidity of the vagina and thereby increase the likelihood that the male sperm cells will survive and be able to get through the usually acid vaginal barrier and into the uterus and finally the tube to impregnate the waiting egg. Dr. Shettles also believes that if the woman has an orgasm before the man does, the female orgasm contributes to the alkalinity of the vaginal vault and helps enhance the likelihood of having a boy child. Finally, he recommends that sexual intercourse be done in such a way that the pool of semen is deposited at the innermost end of the vaginal canal at the mouth of the cervix to facilitate rapid entrance of the male sperm cells through the cervix into the uterus.

If the couple wants a girl child, they should have inter-

340

course for two or three days before ovulation and then stop at the actual time of ovulation. Moreover, before each act of intercourse the woman can take a slightly acid douche, composed of a couple of tablespoons of white vinegar in a quart of water. It is desirable for the man to have his orgasm without the woman reaching a climax to enhance the acidity of the vaginal vault which will act as a barrier to the male sperm cells and increase the likelihood that the egg will be fertilized with a female sperm cell. The doctor claims 80 percent success with this method.

Dear Dr. Lamb—Would you please settle some friendly arguments for me? Can one ovary or one testicle produce both sexes? Is it the eggs from the ovaries that decide what the sex is to be or is it the sperm from one of the testicles? What are the vitamins required for the testicles to produce sufficient, healthy sperm? Does the size of the testicles have any bearing on their performance? I have heard that a male with only one testicle has a never-ending sperm emission and sex desire. Is this true?

Comment—The sex of the baby is determined by whether a sperm cell from the man that fertilizes the egg has an X chromosome (for female babies) or a Y chromosome (for male babies). Either testicle produces both X and Y sperm. The ovaries do not have anything to do with the sex determination of the baby. It is not true, as some people have asked me, that boys come from one ovary and girls from the other ovary. Also, it is not true that boys come from one testicle and girls from the other testicle.

Generally speaking, the size of the testicles is not important in relation to the man's performance. Small testicles that produce lots of male hormone can cause a man to be sexually very active, even if he happens to be sterile, and having only one testicle certainly doesn't increase a man's sexual performance. If it did, there would be a lot of men going to have one removed. Vitamin A deficiency can cause sterility in the male, but all vitamins are important.

341

GRUNTING AND GROANING

Dear Dr. Lamb—I must ask you a sensitive question. I am a young seventy-eight-year-old woman and a widow. I rent two apartments in my home. A few years ago I had a full-grown woman who made noises like whining and groaning during the night. They were having intercourse. It was so bad that I lost another good tenant because of the disturbance.

I have rented to several newly married couples and never again experienced anything like it until recently. This new couple has been married about two months. I seldom get a night's rest because of her whining and moaning. Is it possible that intercourse can be such a painful experience? I am at my wit's end. Would Vaseline help? I think it is uncalled for. Can you help me before I have a nervous breakdown? I don't know how to handle this situation.

Comment—There are a number of people who are noisy lovers. They express their excitement with the sex act by grunting, groaning, and making verbal comments. This habit is called erolalia. Some people claim it relaxes them during the sex act and helps to increase their enjoyment. It does not mean that either one of the sex partners is in pain, merely that they are getting carried away with the act and thoroughly enjoying it. It frequently does cause complaints of "what will the neighbors think," particularly for apartment-dwellers. I suppose one solution to this lady's problem, since she's the landlord, is to soundproof the couple's bedroom and wear earmuffs to bed.

INDEX

Abortion, 96-100
Acton, William, 4
Acute prostatitis, 297
Adrenal glands, 224
Alcohol, 161-62, 167
Amazons, 5
Anemia, 50
Anti-sex women, 282-86
Artificial insemination, 115-16
Aspirin, sterility and, 330-31
Atchek, Albert, 102
Atherosclerosis, 111, 154, 273
Atrophic vaginitis, 279, 288

Babies, predetermining sex of, 339-41
Balding, 78
Bestiality, 41
Benedek, Thomas, 166
Bent penis, 196-97
Biller, Henry, 140
Birth control, 65-100
    abortion and, 96-100
    creams and foams, 91-92
    diaphragm and, 94-95
    female sterilization, 67-72
    IUD, 92-94
    male sterilization, 72-78

pills, 82-91
    rhythm method, 78-82
    withdrawal, 95-96
Bisexuality, 139-40
Bladder, 65, 73, 244-45
    prostate and, 262, 263, 266
Bleeding, 254-55
Body temperature, 80-81
Boys
    homosexuality and, 145-46
    masturbation and, 125-27
Brassiere, use of, 213-14
Breasts, 37, 205-23
    cancer of, 216-21, 233-34
    discharge, 214-15
    of men, 221-23
    nipples, 216
    pains in, 214
    size of, 206-14
Burch, John, 234
Busse, William F., 81
Byra, Benjamin, 234

Caesar, Julius, 138-39
Calderwood, Deryck, 8
Calhoun, David W., 86
Cancer, vaginal, 329-30
Cancer of the breasts, 216-21
    menopause hormone therapy and, 233-34

Cancer of the prostate, 264-65
Cancers and tumors, 252-56
Carlson, Hjalmar, 77
Cartwright, Ann, 66
Castration, 268-69, 271
Cervix, 67, 82, 193, 230
  cancer of, 253-55
  herniation of, 246
  hysterectomy and, 246-51
  vaginal discharge and, 217
Cesarean section, 331-32
Chalon, Jack, 234
Chest, 221-23
Childbirth, cesarean section and, 331-32
Chopin, Frédéric, 140
Christ, Takey, 66
Chronic mastitis, 215, 221
Cicero, 138
Circumcision, 197-200
Clinical Pharmacology and Therapeutics, 268
Clitoral orgasm, 31
Clitoris, 43-44
Clotting, birth control pills and, 86-87
Community Sex Information Education Service (New York), 2
Condoms, 85, 307-308
Corpus luteum, 83
Crab lice, 312-13
Cramps, menstrual, 53-56
Cream, birth control, 91-92
Cryptorchidism, 200
Cystitis, 64-65, 189, 245

Cystocele, 244-45, 246
Cystoscopy, 263
Cysts of the breasts, 220

da Vinci, Leonardo, 152
Davis, Catherine B., 117, 121
DeBrouner, Charles H., 68
Desire
  frequency of sex and, 273-76
  lack of, 173-80
Diabetes, 155, 186
Diaphragm, 94-95
Dickes, Robert, 325-26
Dickinson, Robert, 15, 118, 120, 187, 192
Dilatation and curettage (D&C), 105, 247, 254, 256
Diminished fluids, 276-79
Discharge and hygiene, 287-92
  vaginal discharges, 290-92
  vulva, 288-90
Discharges, 249-51
Discharges of the breasts, 214-15
Dorval, Marie, 140
Douching, 47, 59-62, 287
"Drag queens," 318
Drill, Victor, 86
Drugs, 333-34
Dysmenorrhea, 54
Dyspareunia, 187-90

Electrocautery, 263
Endocrine glands, 20
Endometriosis, 251-52
Endometrium, cancer of,

255-56
Epididymis, 264
Epididymitis, 203
Erectile tissue, 205
Erections, 327-29
  failure of, 152-68
Estrogen, 32, 83-84, 211,
  278-79
  menopause and, 226, 227,
  234

Facial hair, 226
Fainting, 57-58
Family planning, 66
Female sexual dysfunctions,
  173-90
  lack of desire, 173-80
  orgasm failure, 180-87
  painful intercourse, 187-90
Female sterilization, 67-72
Female surgery, 242-56
  cancers and tumors, 252-56
  endometriosis, 251-52
  stretched pelvic muscles,
  242-46
  virginity and, 246-51
Feminine hygiene deodorants,
  287-89
Fetishism, 321-26
Fibroadenosis, 215, 221
Fibroid tissues, 252-53
Fink, Paul, 143
Flagyl, 291
Fluid accumulation, 57-58
Foam, birth control, 91-92
  venereal disease and, 84
Follicle-stimulating

hormone (FSH), 83-84
Foreskin, 197-200
Foster, Raymond O., 81
Freedman, Daniel X., 317-18
Frequency of sex, 18-26
  desire and, 273-76
Freud, Sigmund, 9, 135, 325
Frigidity, 44, 173
Fungus, vaginal, 288, 291-92

Gandhi, Mohandas, 5-6
Garcia, Celso-Raymon, 107
Ginsberg, George L., 153
Girls
  homosexuality and, 146-48
  masturbation and, 119-22
Gonorrhea, 2, 39, 41, 107, 288,
  294-301
Graham, Billy, 8
Gravelee, L. Clark, 256
Greece, 138
Gregg, Allen, 12
Grimes, John W., 330
Grunting and groaning, 342

Hair loss, 331
Hammond, William, 4
Hastings, Donald, 182
Heart disease, sex and,
  334-38
Hernias, 203-204, 245-46
Hoffa, Jimmy, 140
Hoffman, Martin, 141
Homosexuality, 41, 125,
  134-51
  in boys, 145-46
  in girls, 146-48

transvestism and, 318
venereal disease and, 310
wives and, 148-50
Honeymoon cystitis, 64-65,
189
Hormones, 20, 23, 34
birth control pills and,
83-84
menopause therapy with,
230-34
prostate and, 267-69
Hot flashes, 225
Human Sex Anatomy
(Dickinson), 15, 118, 120,
187, 192
Hydroceles, 203-204
Hygiene, discharges and,
287-92
vaginal discharge, 290-92
vulva, 288-90
Hymen, 13-17, 63, 190
hysterectomy and, 246-51
Hyperventilation, 57-58
Hysterectomy, 174, 230,
246-51
Pap test and, 255

Impotence, 152-72, 275-76
erection failure, 152-68
orgasm failure, 171-72
premature ejaculation,
168-71
Intercourse, painful female,
187-90
Intrauterine device (IUD),
92-94

Johnson, Virginia E., 2, 141
on alcoholic impotency,
161
on female orgasm, 31, 54,
120, 180-81
orgasm failure technique
of, 181-82, 184
on penis size, 192
premature ejaculation
technique of, 168-70
on size of vaginal canal,
58, 94
Judaism, 134

K-Y lubricant, 278
Kaye, Bernard, 289, 90
Kettener, Warren A., 310
Kinsey, Alfred, 30, 43, 117,
122, 274
on fetishism, 325
on homosexuality, 134-38,
144, 146
Kolodny, Robert, 186
Kwell, 313

Laparoscopy tubal
sterilization, 71
Ledick, Leonard, 334
Leonardo da Vinci, 152
Leukoplakia, 282
Leukorrhea, 47
Lief, Harold, 118
Little, William, 71
Loew, Dolores, 234
Lorinoz, Albert B., 81
LSD, 334

Lumps on the breasts, 216-21
Lutinizing hormone (LH), 83

McGee, Sylvester, 273
McLeon, Peter J., 268
Maimonides, Moses, 7, 166
Male anatomy problems,
   191-204
  bent penis, 196-97
  circumcision, 197-200
  inflammation of the
    testicles, 203
  penis size, 191-96
  swelling and lumps,
    203-204
  undescended testicles,
    200-201
  varicocele, 201-202
Male breasts, 221-23
Male impotence, *see*
  Impotence
Male masturbation, 125-28
Male menopause, 239-41
Male sterilization, 72-78
Mammography, 217
Margolese, Sidney, 141
Marijuana, 333
Mastectomy, 218
Mastitis, chronic, 215, 221
Masturbation, 117-33
  boys, 125-27
  girls, 119-22
  in marriage, 128-33
  men, 127-28
  older women, 122-23, 274
Masters, William H., 2, 141

  on alcoholic impotence,
    161
  on female orgasm, 31,
    54, 120, 180-81
  orgasm failure technique
    of, 181-82, 184
  on penis size, 192
  premature ejaculation
    technique of, 168-70
  on size of vaginal canal,
    58, 94
Medical World News, 289
Medrogestrone, 268
Menopause, female, 22, 68,
   224-39
  hormone therapy and,
    230-34
  hysterectomy and, 249
  menopausal menses,
    234-36
  pregnancy and, 236-39
  symptoms of, 225-30, 279
Menopause, male, 239-41
Menstrual cycle, 32-35, 38
Menstruation, 16, 47-53, 84,
   103-104
  cramps of, 53-56
  hygiene during, 59
  menopausal menses,
    234-36
  premenstrual tension,
    56-57
  sex during, 58-59
Miscarriage, 27-28
Mojave Indians, 138
Monilia, 288, 291-92

Morning sickness, 38
Mucus, 82
Mumps, 113-14, 203

Nero, 5
New Guinea, 4
Nipples, 216, 219
Nonspecific urethritis, 296
Nymphomania, 28-29

Odor, 39-40, 287
Ogilvie, R. I., 268
Old age, sex and, 272-86
  anti-sex women, 282-86
  desire and frequency,
    273-76
  diminished fluids, 276-79
  sex after surgery, 279-81
  sex variety, 281-82
Oral-genital sex, 38-43, 281,
  289
Orgasm, 31, 273
  orgasm failure, 171-72,
    180-87
Orkin, Louis, 234
Ovaries, 67, 83-84, 341
Ovulation, 33-34, 83-84, 103
  menopause and, 224
  ovulatory pain and, 48
Ovum, 32

Pacion, Stanley, 138
Painful intercourse,
  female, 187-90
Pains in breasts, 214
Pap test, 253-56
Pelvic muscles, stretched,
    242-46
Penis, 73
  bent, 196-97
  circumcision of, 197-200
  size of, 191-96
Pessary, 245
Peterson, James A., 272
Peyronie's disease, 196-97
Pills, birth control, 82-91, 211-12
  menopause and, 232-33,
    239-40
Pituitary gland, 83, 225
Playboy, 332-33
Plutarch, 139
Polatin, Philip, 180
Pompeia, 139
Pregnancy, 16
  douching and, 60-61
  fertile period for, 32-37
  intercourse and, 26-28
  menopause and, 236-39
  menstrual flow and, 52
  signs of, 37-38
  venereal disease and,
    297-98
  See also Birth control
Premature ejaculation,
  168-71
Premenstrual tension, 56-57
Procreation, 8
Progesterone, 83-84
Prolapsed uterus, 244
Prostatitis, 297, 330
Prostitution, 6-7
Prostate gland, 36, 73, 156
    257-71, 296-97
  cancer of, 264-65

hormones and, 267-69
operations on, 263-64,
  280-81
postoperative problems
  of, 265-67
prevention of trouble with,
  269-71
symptoms of trouble with,
  258-63
testosterone and, 240-41
Puberty, 194, 222
Puttkamer, Jesco Von, 5

Radical mastectomy, 218
Rangno, Robert E., 268
Rectal sex, 39, 40-41
Rectocele, 246, 250
Rectum, 243-44
Redlich, Frederick C., 317-18
Rhythm method of birth
  control, 78-82
Rome, 138-39
Ruedy, John, 268

Saliva test for ovulation,
  81-82
Sand, George, 140, 320
Scrotum, 73
Semen, 73, 110
  bloody, 330
Seminal vessicle, 36, 73-74,
  257-58, 330
Senile vaginitis, 279, 282
Sensuous Woman, The, 185
Serum acid phosphatase, 265
Sex education, 8
Sexual mores, 3-8

Shettles, Landrum, 339-40
Silicone injections, 207-208
Smegma, 199
Smith, David E., 139
Sparta, 138
Sperm, 36, 73
Spermatoceles, 203-204
Spirochete, 302
Spotting, 33, 38, 51
Sterility, 101-16
  aspirin and, 331
Sterilization, 67-78
Stilbestrol, 226, 329
"Stonies," 202
Surgery, sex after, 279-81
Syphilis, 2, 39, 302-306

Tampons, 62-64
Tension, premenstrual, 56-57
Testicles, 73, 111, 114, 154,
  273
  cancer of, 334
  inflammation of, 203
  male menopause and, 224,
    240
  removal of, 268-69, 271
  undescended, 200-201
  varicocele, 114, 201-202
Testosterone, 73, 112, 141,
  164, 240, 268-69
*Theory and Practice of
  Psychiatry* (Redlich and
  Freedman), 317-18
Thermography, 216, 219
Trahey, Jane, 314
Transurethral resection, 263
Transvestism, 314-21

Trichomoniasis, 288, 290-92
Twins, 339

Undescended testicles,
  200-201
Unitarian Church, 8
Unwed mothers, 2
Urethra, 65, 73, 120, 187, 296
Urethral tube, 102, 257-58,
  262, 263
Urine, 73
Uterine contractions, 28
Uterus, 32-33, 37, 67
  endometriosis, 251-52,
    255-56
  fibroid tumors, 252-53
  hysterectomy and, 248
  menopause and, 230
  stretched pelvic muscles
    and, 242-46

Vagina, 15, 82, 120-22
  cancer of, 329-30
  double, 339
  douching and, 59-62
  hygiene of, 287-92
  lubrication of, 277-79
  stretched muscles of, 161,
    229-30, 242-46
  tampons, 62-64
  venereal disease and, 294
Vaginal discharge, 45-47
Vaginal orgasm, 31
Vaginal stenosis, 102
Vaginitis, atrophic, 279, 288
Variococele, 114, 201-202
Variety, sex, 38-43, 281-82
Vas deferens, 73
Vasectomy, 72-78

prostate and, 269
Venereal disease, 2, 30, 39,
  41, 84, 221, 293-313
  douching and, 60
  gonorrhea, 294-301
  syphilis, 302-306
Virginity, 13-18
  surgery and, 246-51
Vulva, 288-90
Vulvitis, 288-89

Weight gain, 227
Wet dreams, 29-31, 159-60
Withdrawal, 95-96
Women, 45-65
  anti-sex, 282-86
  believed sexless, 4
  cramps, 53-56
  douching, 59-62
  fainting, 57-58
  honeymoon cystitis, 64-65
  hygiene during periods, 59
  masturbation, 119-23
  menstruation, 47-53
  normal discharge, 45-47
  premenstrual tension,
    56-57
  sex during periods, 58-59
  tampons, 62-64
  See also Breasts; Female
    sexual dysfunction;
    Female surgery;
    Menopause, female
Women's Liberation
  Movement, 153
Wulson, John, 213

Yeast infection, vaginal,
  288, 291-92